Problems for Biomedical Fluid Mechanics and Transport Phenomena

How does one deal with a moving control volume? What is the best way to make a complex biological transport problem tractable? Which principles need to be applied to solve a given problem? How do you know whether your answer makes sense?

This unique resource provides over 200 well-tested biomedical engineering problems that can be used as classroom and homework assignments, quiz material, and exam questions. Questions are drawn from a wide range of topics, covering fluid mechanics, mass transfer, and heat transfer applications. These problems, which are motivated by the philosophy that mastery of biotransport is learned by practice, will aid students in developing the key skills of determining which principles to apply and how to apply them.

Each chapter starts with basic problems and progresses to more difficult questions. Lists of material properties, governing equations, and charts provided in the appendices make this book a fully self-contained resource. Solutions to problems are provided online for instructors.

Mark Johnson is Professor of Biomedical Engineering, Mechanical Engineering, and Ophthalmology at Northwestern University. He has made substantial contributions to the study of the pathogenesis of glaucoma and of age-related macular degeneration of the retina. His academic interests include biofluid and biotransport issues, especially those related to ocular biomechanics.

C. Ross Ethier holds the Lawrence L. Gellerstedt, Jr. Chair in Bioengineering and is a Georgia Research Alliance Eminent Scholar in Biomechanics and Mechanobiology at Georgia Tech and Emory University. His academic interests include cell and tissue biomechanics and mechanobiology. He is co-author of *Introductory Biomechanics: From Cells to Organisms*, one of the Cambridge Texts in Biomedical Engineering.

CAMBRIDGE TEXTS IN BIOMEDICAL ENGINEERING

Series Editors
W. Mark Saltzman, Yale University
Shu Chien, University of California, San Diego

Series Advisors
Jerry Collins, Alabama A & M University
Robert Malkin, Duke University
Kathy Ferrara, University of California, Davis
Nicholas Peppas, University of Texas, Austin
Roger Kamm, Massachusetts Institute of Technology
Masaaki Sato, Tohoku University, Japan
Christine Schmidt, University of Texas, Austin
George Truskey, Duke University
Douglas Lauffenburger Massachusetts Institute of Technology

Cambridge Texts in Biomedical Engineering provide a forum for high-quality textbooks targeted at undergraduate and graduate courses in biomedical engineering. It covers a broad range of biomedical engineering topics from introductory texts to advanced topics, including biomechanics, physiology, biomedical instrumentation, imaging, signals and systems, cell engineering, and bioinformatics, as well as other relevant subjects, with a blending of theory and practice. While aiming primarily at biomedical engineering students, this series is also suitable for courses in broader disciplines in engineering, the life sciences and medicine.

Problems for Biomedical Fluid Mechanics and Transport Phenomena

Mark Johnson
Northwestern University, Illinois

C. Ross Ethier
Georgia Institute of Technology and Emory University

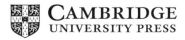
CAMBRIDGE
UNIVERSITY PRESS

CAMBRIDGE
UNIVERSITY PRESS

University Printing House, Cambridge CB2 8BS, United Kingdom

Published in the United States of America by Cambridge University Press, New York

Cambridge University Press is part of the University of Cambridge.

It furthers the University's mission by disseminating knowledge in the pursuit of education, learning, and research at the highest international levels of excellence.

www.cambridge.org
Information on this title: www.cambridge.org/9781107037694

© M. Johnson and C. R. Ethier 2014

First published 2014

Printed and bound in the United States of America

A catalog record for this publication is available from the British Library

ISBN 978-1-107-03769-4 Hardback

Additional resources for this publication at www.cambridge.org/johnsonandethier

To my wife, son, parents, and family,
and to my mentors, colleagues, and students,
who have all in their own ways contributed to this book
Mark Johnson

To my students, colleagues, and family,
who have all taught me so much.
C. Ross Ethier

"A tremendously valuable resource for bioengineering students and instructors that contains problems scaling from the molecular to whole body level. Nearly every system in the body is included, as well as a variety of clinically and industrially relevant situations. The problems are aimed at instruction in applying basic physical principles in a variety of settings, and include entertaining topics such as squid swimming, elephant ear heat transfer, whistling to spread germs, and air friction over a bicyclist. What fun!"

James E. Moore Jr., Imperial College London

"The problems and solutions represent an invaluable resource for instructors. In addition, the step-by-step procedure described in section 1.3 is a wonderfully insightful reminder of what students really need to know to be successful in solving fluid mechanics problems. Instructors would do well to teach this procedure at the beginning and to refer to it consistently throughout the course."

M. Keith Sharp, University of Louisville

"A book devoted solely to biologically relevant problems in fluid mechanics and transport is a very welcome addition to the teaching armamentarium in this area. Problems related to cardiovascular, respiratory and ocular physiology are emphasized, deriving from the substantial research expertise of the authors. The problems are very interesting and in many cases very challenging. They cover a range of difficulty that should be appropriate for both undergraduate and graduate level courses and more than enough topics to provide substantial breadth. Overall excellent! Now I'm looking forward to working out my own solutions and maybe peeking at the solution manual."

John M. Tarbell, The City College of New York

Contents

Preface

This book arose out of a need that frequently faced us, namely coming up with problems to use as homework in our classes and to use for quizzes. We have found that many otherwise excellent textbooks in transport phenomena are deficient in providing challenging but basic problems that teach the students to apply transport principles and learn the crucial engineering skill of problem solving. A related challenge is to find such problems that are relevant to biomedical engineering students.

The problems included here arise from roughly the last 20–30 years of our collective teaching experiences. Several of our problems have an ancestry in a basic set of fluid mechanics problems first written by Ascher Shapiro at MIT and later extended by Ain Sonin, also at MIT. Roger Kamm at MIT also generously donated some of his problems that are particularly relevant to biomedical transport phenomena. Thanks are due to Zdravka Cankova and Nirajan Rajkarnikar, who helped with proof-reading of the text and provided solutions for many of the problems.

For the most part, the problems in this book do not involve detailed mathematics or theoretical derivations. Nor do they involve picking a formula to use and then plugging in numbers to find an answer. Instead, most of the problems presented require skills in problem solving. That is, much of the challenge in these problems involves deciding how to approach them and what principle or principles to apply.

Students will need to understand how to pick a control volume, and that multiple control volumes are necessary for some problems. How does one deal with a moving control volume? How many principles need to be applied to solve a given problem? How do you know whether your answer makes sense? Students who are struggling or stuck on a particular problem will want to know how they should proceed in such cases. The problems presented here will raise all of these issues for students.

In the first chapter, we give general principles of problem solving, and present the Reynolds transport theorem. We also show an example of how we would approach and solve one problem. However, problem solving is best learned by doing problems. Seeing someone else solve a problem is not nearly as educational. We hope that we have provided a wide variety of problems in different areas of transport phenomena, most at the basic level, that aids in the development of problem-solving skills for students in these areas. Each chapter of problems is organized such that the easier problems are at the beginning of the chapter, and then the problems become progressively harder. The exception to this rule is that heat transfer problems are to be found at the end of each chapter.

1 Problem solving

In this introductory chapter, we begin with a derivation of the Reynolds transport theorem, which is central to conservation principles applied to control volumes. Then, we turn to the issue of how to approach problem solving.

1.1 The Reynolds transport theorem

Quantities, such as mass, momentum, energy and even entropy and money, are conserved in the sense that the following principle can be applied to a system.

Input + Generation = Output + Accumulation

The system normally considered in transport phenomena for application of this principle is a control volume. The equation makes intuitive sense and is simple to apply in many cases. However, when moving control volumes and reference frames are examined, or when transport of quantities that have direction (such as momentum) is considered, intuition is less reliable. We here derive a rigorous version of this conservation principle and, in the process, discover the wide applicability of the Reynolds transport theorem. We note that more intuitive formulations of this principle can be found in other texts (e.g. *Fluid Mechanics* by Potter and Foss).

We consider a generalization of Leibniz's rule for the differentiation of integrals. Consider a given function[1] $f(x)$ and the definite integral (M) of this function between $x = a$ and $x = b$. Let both this function and the limits of integration be functions of time (t) (see the figure):

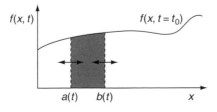

---

[1] Note that f could be either a scalar- or a vector-valued function. We write it here as a scalar (unbolded).

$$M = \int_{a(t)}^{b(t)} f(x,t)dx$$

Using the chain rule, we can find how the value of this integral changes with time:

$$\frac{dM}{dt} = \frac{\partial M}{\partial t} + \frac{\partial M}{\partial a}\frac{da}{dt} + \frac{\partial M}{\partial b}\frac{db}{dt}$$

or

$$\frac{dM}{dt} = \int_{a(t)}^{b(t)} \frac{\partial f(x,t)}{\partial t}dt + f[b(t),t]\frac{db}{dt} - f[a(t),t]\frac{da}{dt}$$

This is Leibniz's rule, which is well known from calculus. M changes with time not only due to temporal changes in f, but also because the boundaries of integration move. Note that the temporal derivative was taken inside the integral, since a and b are held constant in the partial derivative. This will be important when we consider moving control volumes.

We now look to apply a similar principle but in three dimensions, relating the time rate of change of a moving system to that of a stationary system. This is particularly important in transport phenomena, not simply because our systems are frequently moving, but, more importantly, because our laws of physics are derived for material volumes, not control volumes.

A material volume is a fixed, identifiable set of matter.[2] A control volume is a region of space, fixed or moving, that we choose to analyze. Our laws of physics apply directly to matter, not to control volumes. For example, physics tells us that (for non-relativistic systems) mass is conserved. Thus, the mass of a given material volume is always constant. But the mass in a control volume can change.

Solving a problem by tracking the moving material volume is known as a Langrangian approach. It is typically quite difficult to solve problems in this way since material volumes change their location and shape due to their motion. Analysis is facilitated by use of a control volume whose shape and motion can be specified; such an approach is known as Eulerian. However, to use an Eulerian approach, we require the Reynolds transport theorem, which allows us to relate physical laws that are derived for material volumes to a principle that applies to

---

[2] Also referred to by some authors as a "control mass." Note that the use of the term "fixed" in the above definition does not imply that the material volume is not moving; rather, it means that its constituent parts are neither destroyed nor created, although they can be transformed into other components through e.g. chemical reactions.

control volumes. In other words, the Reynolds transport theorem acts as a "bridge" between material volumes, where the physical laws are defined, and control volumes, which are more convenient for analysis.

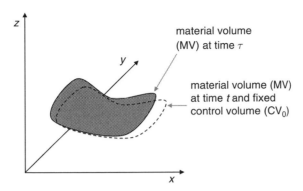

Consider a moving material volume as shown in the figure above. This material volume is moving such that it occupies the region surrounded by the dashed line at time t and the solid line at a later time τ. Note that the points within the material volume are not all necessarily moving with the same velocity (e.g. a fluid or a deforming solid).

Pick a control volume that coincides with the material volume at time t. We define M as the integral of a function $f(x, t)$ over the material volume,

$$M = \int_{MV} f(\boldsymbol{x}, t) d\boldsymbol{x}$$

where $\boldsymbol{x} = (x, y, z)$. We will relate M to the integral of the same function, $f(\boldsymbol{x}, t)$, over the control volume.

We use an analogous approach to that leading to Leibniz's equation. We consider the integral of a function $f(\boldsymbol{x}, t)$ over the material volume. M changes with time due both to temporal changes in $f(\boldsymbol{x}, t)$ and to the motion of the boundary of the domain of integration. Noting that the final two terms in Leibniz's equation arise due to the flux of f at the boundary carried by the material's velocity out of the control volume (and thus normal to the control surface), we find that the three-dimensional equivalent of Leibniz's equation becomes

$$\frac{dM}{dt} = \int_{CV_0} \frac{\partial f(\boldsymbol{x}, t)}{\partial t} d\boldsymbol{x} + \int_{CS_0} f(\boldsymbol{x}, t) \left(\vec{V}_{MV} \cdot \hat{n} \right) dS$$

where CS_0 is the surface surrounding the control volume CV_0, $\vec{V}_{MV}$ is the velocity of the material volume, and $\hat{n}$ is the outward pointing unit normal.

This is the Reynolds transport theorem for a stationary control volume. It relates the time rate of change of an intensive function, f (a parameter per unit volume), integrated over a material volume to the integral of that intensive function integrated over a control volume. The second integral over the control surface involves the flux of material entering or leaving the control volume. Note that no material enters or leaves a material volume (by definition).

It is frequently convenient when solving transport problems to consider moving control volumes. To generalize the Reynolds transport theorem, consider both a stationary control volume CV_0 and a control volume CV moving at velocity $\vec{V}_{CV}$, and their respective surfaces, CS_0 and CS (see the figure below).

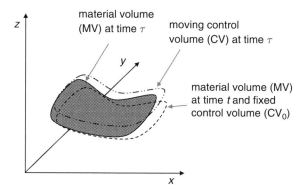

Now, to find the generalized Reynolds transport theorem for the moving control volume, we use the Reynolds transport theorem twice: the first time relating the moving material volume to the stationary control volume, and the second time relating the moving control volume to the stationary control volume:

$$\frac{d}{dt}\int_{MV} f(x,t)dx = \int_{CV_0} \frac{\partial f(x,t)}{\partial t}dx + \int_{CS_0} f(x,t)\left(\vec{V}_{MV} \cdot \hat{n}\right)dS$$

$$\frac{d}{dt}\int_{CV} f(x,t)dx = \int_{CV_0} \frac{\partial f(x,t)}{\partial t}dx + \int_{CS_0} f(x,t)\left(\vec{V}_{CV} \cdot \hat{n}\right)dS$$

On subtracting the second equation from the first, rearranging, and evaluating at time t when the two control volumes are coincident (so that CS and CS_0 are identical), we find

$$\frac{d}{dt}\int_{MV} f(\mathbf{x},t)d\mathbf{x} = \frac{d}{dt}\int_{CV} f(\mathbf{x},t)d\mathbf{x} + \int_{CS} f(\mathbf{x},t)\left(\overrightarrow{V}_{rel}\cdot\hat{n}\right)dS$$

where $\overrightarrow{V}_{rel}$ is the velocity of the material volume relative to the moving control volume. This is the general form of the Reynolds transport theorem, and it is valid for stationary and moving control volumes.

The physical interpretation of this equation is useful. This is a conservation law for any conserved quantity f, in which f is an intensive variable (expressed per unit volume). The term on the left-hand side of the equation is the rate at which f is generated. The first term on the right-hand side of the equation is the accumulation term: the rate at which f accumulates in the control volume. The final term is the flux term, characterizing the balance of the flux of f out of and into the control volume due to flow. Thus, the Reynolds transport theorem recovers our initial conservation principle, namely

Generation = Accumulation + Output − Input

1.2   Application of the Reynolds transport theorem

By applying the laws of physics to the left-hand side of this equation, conservation laws that apply to control volumes can be generated. For example, when considering mass conservation, the function f becomes the fluid density ρ (mass per unit volume, an intensive variable). Then the left-hand side of the equation is simply the time rate of change of the mass of the material volume. Since this mass is constant (mass is not generated), we find that

$$0 = \frac{d}{dt}\int_{CV} \rho(\mathbf{x},t)d\mathbf{x} + \int_{CS} \rho(\mathbf{x},t)\left(\overrightarrow{V}_{rel}\cdot\hat{n}\right)dS$$

This is the mass-conservation equation, which is valid for all non-relativistic control volumes, indicating that accumulation in a control volume results from an imbalance between the influx and outflow of mass from a control volume.

For species conservation, we let $f = C_i$ (moles of species i per unit volume). There are two important differences from the law of mass conservation. First, there is the possibility of generation or destruction of species i due to chemical reactions. We will let the net generation rate of species i be Ψ_i, i.e. the production rate minus the destruction rate. Second, in addition to the flow carrying species i ($C_i\overrightarrow{V}_{rel}$), the diffusion of this species needs to be accounted for.

The diffusional flux of species i is given by Fick's law of diffusion[3]: $\overrightarrow{j_i} = -D_i\nabla C_i$, where D_i is the diffusion coefficient of species i. Taking the dot

---

[3] For isothermal, isobaric conditions.

product of this vector with the unit outward normal to the control surface and integrating over the control surface gives the total net diffusional transport out of the control volume. We then use the Reynolds transport theorem to find the species conservation equation:

$$\int_{CV} \Psi_i(\mathbf{x}, t)\,d\mathbf{x} = \frac{d}{dt}\int_{CV} C_i(\mathbf{x}, t)\,d\mathbf{x} + \int_{CS} C_i(\mathbf{x}, t)\left(\overrightarrow{V}_{rel} \cdot \hat{n}\right) dS$$

$$+ \int_{CS} (\overrightarrow{J_i}(\mathbf{x}, t) \cdot \hat{n})\,dS$$

Likewise, if we allow that $f = \rho \overrightarrow{V}$ (momentum per unit volume, a vector), then the left-hand side of the Reynolds transport theorem is the time rate of change of the momentum of the material volume. This we know from Newton's second law must be the sum of the forces acting on the material volume. Thus, the momentum equation is derived:

$$\sum \overrightarrow{F} = \frac{d}{dt}\int_{CV} \rho\overrightarrow{V}(\mathbf{x}, t)\,d\mathbf{x} + \int_{CS} \rho\overrightarrow{V}(\mathbf{x}, t)\left(\overrightarrow{V}_{rel} \cdot \hat{n}\right) dS$$

This is a vector equation that describes a momentum balance in each of the coordinate directions.

Note that we have imposed no restrictions on the motion of our control volume when deriving the momentum-conservation equation. It can even be accelerating. However, the reference frame (which is not the same as the control volume) cannot be accelerating because Newton's second law does not hold (without modification) for non-inertial reference frames.

Note also that the second integral in the above equation contains two velocities that are not necessarily the same. One is the velocity of the material volume (the fluid), while the other is the relative velocity between the fluid and the control volume. The velocities can even be in different directions (e.g. transferring x-momentum in the y-direction such as might occur when one skater passes another and throws a book in a perpendicular direction that is caught by the slower skater).

The relative velocity in the last term of the momentum equation is present as the dot product with the outward normal, so only the component of $\overrightarrow{V}_{rel}$ that carries material across the control surface contributes to the integral. The sign of a term can be confusing to determine: the sign of any component of $\overrightarrow{V}$ is established by the coordinate direction, e.g. a positive V_x is one that points in the same direction as the x-axis. However, the sign of the term $\overrightarrow{V}_{rel} \cdot \hat{n}$ is determined only by whether fluid is entering or leaving the control volume, being negative or positive, respectively. Students must pay attention to this tricky point!

Application of the Reynolds transport theorem for other parameters can yield equations of angular-momentum conservation or energy conservation. Some of the problems in this book are best tackled using the conservation principles applied to judiciously chosen control volumes.

Unfortunately, many errors are made in applying these principles. Students frequently have difficulties applying the various forms of the Reynolds transport theorem to moving control volumes, especially when vector quantities are involved. The relative velocity that appears in the Reynolds transport theorem is frequently a source of confusion, as noted above.

Students generally have difficulty in approaching transport problems. This is in no small part due to difficulty in thinking in terms of an Eulerian analysis, since much of the physics that students first learn is necessarily taught from a Lagrangian point of view. We now turn to the more general topic of problem solving.

1.3   Approaching transport problems

It is our experience that many students have difficulty with problem solving because they start "in the middle," i.e. write down a conservation law and begin to use it without first deciding **what** they want to conserve and how they should approach the problem. As is the case in so many things in life, it pays to invest some effort in deciding how you want to tackle the problem before diving in. We provide here a set of steps designed to help you make this investment.

1. Draw a GOOD figure. Include all relevant aspects of the problem – the more detailed the figure, the better. Include the physical dimensions of the system and the physical properties of the materials which are given in the problem statement. Decide on sign conventions and a datum (if needed). For example, which direction will be positive and which negative? Where is the origin? (This will be required for use of linear- or angular-momentum conservation. Write the positive directions on your diagram.) Note that, once you have established a positive direction, you have to be consistent: you can't have the x-component of velocity be considered positive rightward but the x-component of force be positive leftward!

Use physical insights to help you characterize the process (e.g. draw streamlines on the figure). List your assumptions. Take some time to do step 1 well, because it is important!

2. Decide what physical law(s) and equation(s) you might want to apply.

- Mass conservation (and, in problems with more than one species, each obeys a conservation principle)
- Linear-momentum conservation and in which direction. Note that linear-momentum conservation cannot be applied in the radial direction (why?).
- Angular-momentum conservation
- Energy conservation
- Bernoulli's equation
- Fick's law of diffusion
- The Navier–Stokes equations
- The convection–diffusion equation

If unsure where to begin, start with application of the simplest law (mass conservation) and progress from there. Students often ask "how do I know what laws to use?" You will learn this by doing problems and gathering experience. Unfortunately, there is no short-cut that substitutes for experience in this case.

3. Pick an object to apply the physical law to. This is a crucial step. This can be a control volume, a free-body diagram, or a streamline (and, if one is applying a differential equation such as the Navier–Stokes equation, a domain must be chosen). Draw this on your figure (don't just visualize it in your head). In the case of a control volume, you **must** give careful consideration to where the boundaries of the volume will lie. You should pick these boundaries according to the "know or want to know" principle: the boundaries should lie either at locations at which your variables are specified or at locations at which you wish to determine the value of a variable. Also, for the application of momentum conservation, avoid cutting any objects with the control surface, since this introduces an unknown force or stress at this location (unless this is the desired result).

If you are going to use a streamline with Bernoulli's equation, you need to choose the location of the starting and ending points of the streamline and draw them onto your diagram. It is difficult to talk about the pressure, velocity, and elevation at point 1 without knowing exactly where point 1 is!

Note that judicious choice of the object you intend to apply a particular physical law to can make problems much easier to solve. However, there is often more than one choice that will lead you to the solution! Some choices might not give you the information you want, or may make it more difficult to solve the problem, but they are not actually wrong. (For example, you could end up proving that $x = x$, which is not useful but at least is not incorrect.) It is better to pick an object and get started, rather than to sit and debate what the best object or principle to use is.

Finally, regarding control volumes, it is necessary to explicitly decide whether the control volume is moving or stationary, and whether it retains the same shape or is deforming with time. Note that the control volume can even be accelerating, although the reference frame must be inertial (not accelerating) in order to allow use of the momentum theorem (unless an altered form of momentum conservation that introduces the inertial accelerations as pseudo-forces is used).

4. Apply equations to your objects. Note that different physical laws can be applied to different objects. Or, the same law can be applied to different objects. Note the total number of equations.

5. Determine the number of unknowns, remembering that some of your unknowns can be vectors that represent two or three unknown values (in two and three dimensions, respectively). Luckily, in such cases the governing equations are also vector-valued. If you have more unknowns than equations, go back to step 2 and pick another principle and another object to apply this principle to.

6. When the number of equations equals the number of unknowns, solve the equations. Identify any boundary conditions and initial conditions that may be needed to solve the equations, and indicate these on your diagram. Make sure that you have a sufficient number of these given the number of equations and the order of any differential equations.

7. When you obtain your solution, check to make sure that it satisfies your assumptions (e.g. that the Reynolds number is within the assumed range, your assumed streamline is a streamline, etc.).

8. Check the units of your answer. If the units are wrong, go backwards one step at a time to find where the units error occurred. This is an extremely important step that many students miss (regardless of how many times they are told). We refer those readers who believe that units are not important, or that they can be "filled in at the end," to the story of the Gimli Glider (see e.g. en.wikipedia.org/wiki/Gimli_Glider) or the Mars Climate Orbiter (en.wikipedia.org/wiki/Mars_Climate_Orbiter).

In this vein, it is also better to leave all equations in symbolic form and not to plug in numbers until the very last step. This not only makes unit checking easier, but also makes your work easier to follow.

9. Check to make sure your answer makes physical sense (e.g. motion in the correct direction, order of magnitude reasonable, boundary conditions satisfied, common-sense check). It's important not to skip this step! It provides closure to the problem, and allows you to understand in physical terms what your solution implies.

1.4   An example

Now, this all seems straightforward enough. Let's see how we use these principles to solve a problem.

Consider the figure shown overleaf: water (density ρ) enters the box from below through a flexible set of bellows at a flow rate Q, passes through the box and then, at

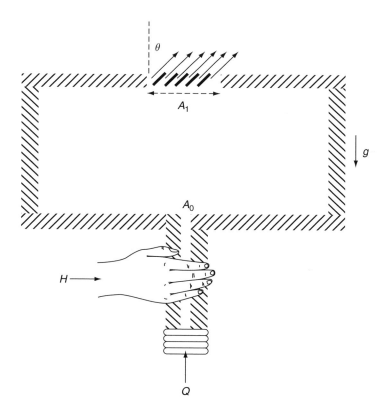

the exit, is directed to the right (at an angle θ) by the slots in the top of the box. We want to find the horizontal force (H) necessary to hold this system stationary under steady-state conditions. We suggest that, before proceeding, you try to work out this problem for yourself.

1. **Draw a good figure**. We begin by re-drawing the figure given in the problem description (do not skip this step), and adding a coordinate system to the figure along with the velocity of the fluid exiting the box. Note that, by observing that we are expressing the velocity of the fluid at the exit as a vector, we now realize that there are two unknowns here.

2. We now decide **what physical laws to apply**. It seems that, if we are to find the force H, then we must apply momentum conservation. However, it is always a good idea to start with mass conservation. This will constrain any answer that we may find, and may give additional insights into the problem.

3. **Pick a control volume**. We know the flow rate Q entering the system at the bottom, so it is useful to have a control surface at this location. Since it will be useful to know the velocity of the fluid leaving the system at the top, it will also be useful to have a control surface at the top of the chamber where the flow leaves the

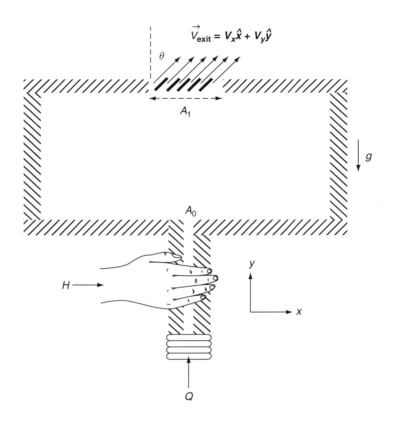

system. The control volume we choose is shown in the figure overleaf as the region surrounded by a dashed line.

4. **Apply equations to object**. We now apply conservation of mass to this control volume.

Since this is a steady-state problem (the time rates of change of all parameters of interest in our problem are zero), the conservation-of-mass equation to apply to this control volume becomes

$$0 = \int_{CS} \rho \left(\vec{V}_{rel} \cdot \hat{n} \right) dS$$

or, simply, inflow equals outflow. But how do we use this simple concept to relate the inflow (Q) to the velocity at the exit?

This surface integral defines this operation. Since $\vec{V}_{rel} = \vec{V}_{fluid} - \vec{V}_{CV}$ and the control volume is stationary, we have that $\vec{V}_{rel} = \vec{V}_{fluid}$. At the surface of this control volume, the fluid velocity is everywhere perpendicular to the unit normal to this surface except at the entrance and exit of the box. Thus,

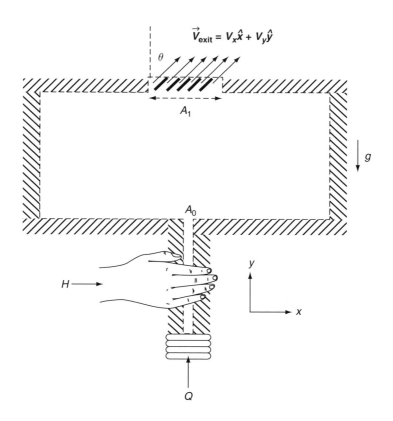

$$0 = \int_{CS_0} \rho \vec{V}_{rel} \cdot \hat{n}\, dS + \int_{CS_1} \rho \vec{V}_{rel} \cdot \hat{n}\, dS$$

where CS_0 is the surface of the control volume at the inlet (area A_0) and CS_1 is that at the exit (area A_1).

Now the first integral is simply $-\rho Q$, the flow entering the system; the negative sign arises because the fluid velocity is in the opposite direction of the outward unit normal to the surface. For the second integral, we need to express $\vec{V}_{rel}$ and $\hat{n}$ as vectors. $\vec{V}_{rel} = \vec{V}_{fluid} = V_x \hat{x} + V_y \hat{y}$ and $\hat{n} = \hat{y}$. Thus, the last integral becomes $\rho v_y A_1$, and we have the result that

$$V_y = \frac{Q}{A}$$

Now we have found one equation describing our system. While not profound, it would have been easy to make a mistake if we had not used the Reynolds transport theorem. Had we been sloppy by setting inflow equal to outflow and letting outflow equal $v_{exit} A_1$ (with v_{exit} as the magnitude of the velocity of the exiting fluid), we would have obtained an incorrect answer. The formalism in the Reynolds transport theorem keeps us on track.

5. **Determine the number of unknowns**. Originally, our unknowns were H (which we want to find) and the two components of the velocity, namely V_x and V_y: three unknowns in total. Since we have found only one equation, we still require two more equations. We return to step 2.

2. **Decide what physical laws to apply**. As expected, we need to apply momentum conservation. Our previous work on mass conservation may make this a little easier. We need not only to decide to apply momentum conservation, but must also decide on a direction to consider. Since our goal is to find H, an x-momentum balance is in order. Thus, we take the x-component of the steady-state momentum equation:

$$\sum F_x = \int_{CS} \rho V_x \left(\vec{V}_{rel} \cdot \hat{n} \right) dS$$

3. **Pick a control volume**. Now we need to pick an object to apply this principle to. Our first choice might be the control volume we picked for mass conservation. However, the question of how we would determine the sum of forces acting in the x-direction on the control volume then arises. The pressure forces inside the flow chamber are unknown, and are not symmetric on the two sides of the control volume (and thus they do not cancel out). Furthermore, this control volume is not directly acted upon by H, and thus the variable of interest will not enter a momentum balance on this CV.

A better choice is shown in the figure overleaf. Although there are pressure forces acting on both sides of this CV (atmospheric pressure), the net pressure force (in the x-direction) cancels out since the pressure acts on this CV symmetrically. Since this CV cuts the hand holding the box, it also introduces the force H. The CV cuts the box only at the flexible bellows (where no force exists due to the flexibility), and thus no other horizontal forces act on this CV.

4. **Apply equations to the object**. Now we apply the x-momentum equation to this CV. Since H is the only net force acting in the x-direction on this CV, we have

$$H = \int_{CS} \rho V_x \left(\vec{V}_{rel} \cdot \hat{n} \right) dS$$

Note that this is now a scalar equation even though it still contains a vector, $\vec{V}_{rel}$. We need to evaluate this integral around the control surface. We have already seen that $\vec{V}_{rel}$ is simply the fluid velocity (since the CV is stationary). The fluid velocity is everywhere perpendicular to the unit normal to the control surface, except at the entrance and the exit. Thus, we need evaluate this integral only at these two locations.

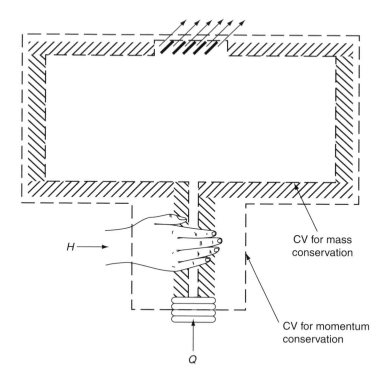

CV for mass
conservation

CV for momentum
conservation

At the entrance, the fluid velocity is entirely in the y-direction, and thus no x-momentum is carried into the CV. The integral thus vanishes on this surface, meaning that it remains only to evaluate the x-momentum flux at the exit:

$$H = \int_{A_1} \rho V_x \left(\overrightarrow{V}_{\text{rel}} \cdot \hat{n} \right) dS$$

Here, we need to find the scalar product $\overrightarrow{V}_{\text{rel}} \cdot \hat{n}$. We showed above (for our mass conservation calculation) that this product is V_y. Thus, we have x-momentum (per unit volume: ρV_x) being carried by the exiting flow in the y-direction (this is the only component of the fluid velocity which is leaving the control volume). This is a non-intuitive result and emphasizes the importance of using the Reynold's transport theorem for solving momentum transport problems.

Thus, we now find that

$$H = \rho V_x V_y A_1$$

5. **Determine the number of unknowns**. We have not introduced any new unknowns, and thus we still have three unknowns. However, we have only two equations, one arising from mass conservation and the other from x-momentum conservation. We need another equation.

While it might seem tempting to now construct a y-momentum balance, this will introduce another unknown, namely the vertical force applied by the hand holding up the box. We could also look for another principle (or a different control volume) to apply.

But it is useful to first examine the known parameters and see whether we have used them all in our analysis. We were given ρ, Q, A_0, A_1, and θ. We have used all of these in our analysis save θ. Since it seems that our answer must depend on θ, we look for another relationship that involves θ.

This we can easily find by noting that the fluid leaves the box at an angle θ. Thus, we see that

$$\frac{V_x}{V_y} = \tan \theta$$

6. **Solve the equations**. On solving these three equations for the force H, we find

$$H = \frac{\rho Q^2 \tan \theta}{A_1}$$

7. **Verify any assumptions**. Since we have used only mass and momentum conservation (which are always valid), we do not have any assumptions to check.

8. **Check units!!** This is such an important step, and so often missed by students. To check units in this case, we take advantage of a little trick. Rewrite the solution in terms of the velocity V_y:

$$H = \rho V_y^2 A_1 \tan \theta$$

Then note that, from Bernoulli's equation, ρV_y^2 must have the same units as pressure. But pressure times area is force. Thus, the units check ($\tan \theta$ is dimensionless).

9. **Check that the answer makes physical sense**. First, check the sign of the answer. The force is positive. Does this make sense? Yes, the momentum from the exiting fluid will force the box to the left. A rightward-directed force must be applied to keep the box in place.

Now look to find a situation where you already know the answer. If θ is zero, then we know that H should be zero (since the exiting fluid is upward). The solution is consistent with this expectation.

Finally, if we increase Q or ρ, H increases. This seems reasonable. If A_1 increases, H decreases. This perhaps is reasonable also, although it is less clear what to expect here. Finally, increasing θ leads to an increased H. This again is what we would expect.

2 Conservation of mass and the Reynolds transport theorem
(11 problems)

2.1. Vascular endothelial cells are cultured on the inside of a 10-cm long hollow tube that has an internal diameter of 3 mm. Culture medium flows through the tube at $Q = 1$ ml/s. The cells produce a cytokine, EDGF, at a rate n_{EDGF} (production rate per cell area) that depends on the local wall shear stress according to $n_{EDGF} = k\tau_{wall}$, where k is an unknown constant with units of ng/dyne per s. The flow in the tube is not fully developed, such that the shear stress is known to vary with axial position according to $\tau_{wall} = \tau_0(1 - \beta x)$, where $\beta = 0.02$ cm^{-1}, $\tau_0 = 19$ dyne/cm^2, and x is the distance from the tube entrance. Under steady conditions a sample of medium is taken from the outlet of the tube, and the concentration of EDGF is measured to be 35 ng/ml in this sample. What is k?

2.2. Flow occurs through a layer of epithelial cells that line the airways of the lung due to a variety of factors, including a pressure difference across the epithelial layer ($\Delta P = P_0$) and, in the case of transient compression, to a change in the separation between the two cell membranes, w_2, as a function of time. We consider these cases sequentially below. Note that the depth of the intercellular space into the paper is L, and the transition in cell separation from w_1 to w_2 occurs over a length δ much smaller than H_1 and H_2. (See the figure overleaf.)

(a) Obtain an expression for U_2, the mean velocity of the fluid exiting from the lower end of the intercellular space ($x = H_1 + H_2$) if fluid is being drawn in (downward) through the cell layer (due to a pressure-driven flow) and into the intercellular space at a rate of q (the rate of flow per unit area of the gap that the fluid is crossing, with the units of q being m^3 s^{-1} m^{-2} or m/s). The widths w_1 and w_2 do not change with time.

(b) Now let $q = 0$, but let w_2 decrease in size at a constant rate $dw_2/dt = -\alpha$. Assume that the width w_2 remains uniform along the entire length of H_2 as w_2 changes. Obtain an expression for the mean velocity of the fluid exiting from the lower end of the intercellular space, $U_2(t)$.

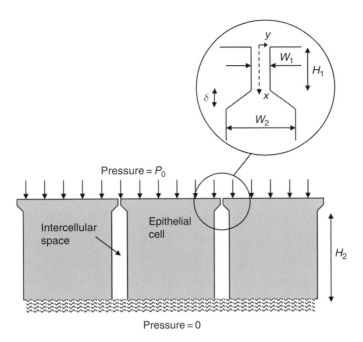

2.3. Consider a capillary of length L and radius R. The hydraulic conductivity is a property that characterizes the rate at which fluid passes through a membrane or other porous structure. It has units of flow rate per unit area per pressure drop. Suppose that the hydraulic conductivity of the capillary wall, L_p, is given by the expression $L_\mathrm{p} = L_\mathrm{p}^0\left(1 + \beta x^k\right)$, where L_p^0, β, and k are constants, and x is the axial position in the capillary, measured from the capillary entrance.

Assume that the pressure drop along the length of the capillary is a linear function of axial position, x, and that the osmotic pressures inside and outside the capillary and the external tissue pressure are all constant. Define the balance point to be the location, x_b, where the local filtration through the capillary wall is zero.

If it is required that there be zero net filtration through the capillary walls, i.e. the net filtration inflow equals the net filtration outflow over the length of the capillary, derive an expression for x_b in terms of the other variables.

2.4. Blood flows in a capillary of uniform radius $R = 10\ \mu\mathrm{m}$ and length $L = 0.1$ cm. Although not strictly true, for the purposes of this problem, we will treat the inlet velocity profile as parabolic:

$$v_x(r) = U_\mathrm{CL}\left[1 - \left(\frac{r}{R}\right)^2\right]$$

with centerline velocity $U_{CL} = 85$ cm/s. Water filters out of the blood and through the capillary wall with filtration velocity u_{filter}:

$$u_{filter} = U_0(1 - ax)$$

with $U_0 = 0.1$ cm/s and $a = 12$ cm^{-1}. This means that water leaves the capillary at the arteriolar end and re-enters at the venular end (Starling's hypothesis). Notice that there is a location at $x = 1/a$ where there is no inflow or outflow of fluid through the artery wall. This is called the balance point.

We are also given that the glucose concentration in the blood entering the capillary is $c_{inlet} = 90$ mg/dl, and the glucose concentration in the resorbed fluid is 30 mg/dl.

(a) Find the average velocity of blood leaving the end of the capillary.
(b) Find the average glucose concentration in the blood at the venular end of the capillary.

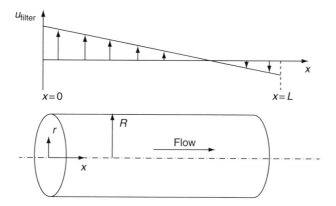

2.5. Fluid flows steadily at flow rate Q through a diverging nozzle with half-angle β, as shown overleaf (only the x-component of velocity is shown). Assume that the v_x velocity profile is given by

$$v_x(x, r) = U_{CL}(x)\left[1 - \left(\frac{r}{R(x)}\right)^2\right]$$

(a) Show that $U_{CL} = 2Q/(\pi R^2)$.
(b) Compute the radial component of velocity, $v_r(x, r)$. Assume incompressible flow.

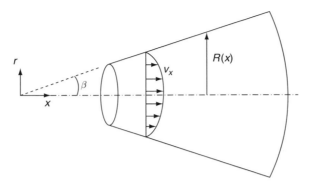

2.6. Blood flow in small vessels has a velocity profile that can be approximated as Poiseuille:

$$v(r) = 2v_{\text{ave}} \left[1 - \left(\frac{r}{R} \right)^2 \right]$$

where R is the vessel radius and r is any radial location. For vessel diameters less than a few hundred micrometers, a curious effect is seen in that the blood hematocrit (volume of red blood cells (RBCs) divided by blood volume) in these vessels is less than the hematocrit in the general circulation. This is called the Fåhræus effect, and is due to the plasma-skimming layer: very near the wall, RBCs are excluded due to their size and their tendency to move away from the wall. The thickness of this layer is approximately 3 μm.

If the hematocrit in the general circulation is 50%, then, assuming that the RBCs are randomly distributed outside of the plasma-skimming layer, what is the "tube hematocrit" (the volume of RBCs in the blood vessel divided by the total blood volume in the same blood vessel) in a blood vessel of diameter 60 μm? You may assume that the "discharge hematocrit," defined as the hematocrit in a blood sample collected at the exit of the vessel, equals the hematocrit in the general circulation. You may also assume a Poiseuille velocity profile.

2.7. When a person goes scuba diving and, after spending time at depth, ascends too quickly, nitrogen bubbles can form in the blood stream. Once formed, these bubbles can grow, and we want to study this process. Assume the density of the gas in the bubble is ρ_1 (gas comes out of solution and into the bubble), while that of the surrounding blood is ρ_2 (ρ_1 and ρ_2 can both be assumed constant). Assume the bubble is growing at a constant velocity v. (You may ignore any movement of the blood except that caused by the expanding bubble.)

(a) Derive an expression for the radial outflow velocity $u(r, t)$ of the blood at a position r from the bubble center for any time t before the arrival of the bubble at r.

(b) The velocity u of the blood right next to the bubble is not equal to v. Explain why in terms of ρ_1 and ρ_2.

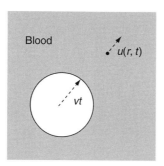

2.8. The eye is mainly filled with vitreous humor and aqueous humor. The vitreous humor is largely stagnant, while the aqueous humor flows into and out of the eye. It enters the eye (from the ciliary processes) at a flow rate of $Q_{in} = 2$ μl/min, and leaves the eye (through the trabecular meshwork) at a flow rate proportional to the intra-ocular pressure (IOP) of the eye: $Q_{out} = (\text{IOP} - P_v)/R$, where P_v is the episcleral venous pressure and R is the flow resistance of the trabecular meshwork. Under normal circumstances, IOP = 15 mm Hg and $P_v = 9$ mm Hg.

The volume of the eye is linearly related to the IOP such that a change in the IOP leads to a change in ocular volume: $\Delta V = C \Delta \text{IOP}$, where C, the compliance of the eye, is approximately 1 μl/mm Hg. Assume that, in a clinical procedure, 20 μl of a therapeutic agent is rapidly injected into the eye (R, C, and P_v remain constant during this process).

(a) Estimate the value to which intraocular pressure in the eye will rise.

(b) Determine how long it will take before the IOP drops to a pressure of 16 mm Hg.

2.9. External pneumatic compression (EPC) is used on bed-ridden patients as one method by which pooling of blood in the legs is prevented. Once a minute, the external pressure (P_e) in a cuff surrounding each lower leg (below the knee) is raised, thus squeezing venous blood out of the lower leg. Let the distance from the foot to the knee be L, and let x be the distance from the foot to any location on the lower leg. To monitor the efficiency of this process, we can use radioactive blood tracers to determine $B(x, t)$, the volume of blood per unit length in the lower leg.

In the following, you may assume that the volume of arterial and capillary blood in the leg remains constant because the pressures used in EPC (less than 50 mm Hg) are too low to affect arterial blood flow.

(a) Find the flow rate of venous blood leaving the lower leg as a function of time during the compression process (you may ignore the steady flow of arterial blood into the leg and the equivalent steady flow of venous blood out of the leg; you may also assume that no blood is squeezed into the foot during the compression process).

(b) Estimate the average velocity of the venous blood in the lower leg as a function of x and t. (For this calculation, you may assume that 75% of the blood in the leg is venous blood.)

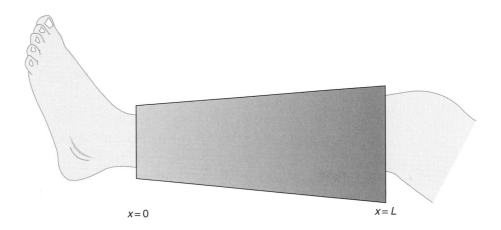

$x=0$ $x=L$

2.10. An experiment is being conducted to investigate the process of chemoattraction of macrophages. A solution of macrophages (n cells per unit volume) is exposed to a chemoattractant. Each of these cells has a density of ρ and a volume of u. This chemoattractant is placed at the center of this solution ($r = 0$). All of the cells move steadily toward $r = 0$ with a velocity (v) that depends on their distance away from the center (r): $v = v_0 r_0^2 / r^2$, where v_0 and r_0 are constants. This causes a growing sphere of cells to accumulate around $r = 0$. The density of this sphere of cells is ρ, the radius of this sphere is $A(t)$, and $A(t = 0) = r_0$.

You may assume that the size of the cells is much smaller than $A(t)$. Find $dA(t)/dt$.

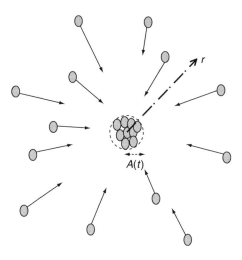

2.11. When considering flow through vessels in the body, such as arteries and veins, the dimensions of the vessels cannot be considered constant but vary with changes in pressure within their lumen. We wish to derive the one-dimensional mass-conservation law for flow in such a vessel.

(a)   Consider the flow of an incompressible fluid through the vessel below and determine the unsteady, one-dimensional differential form of the mass-conservation law for such a vessel, where $u(x, t)$ is the cross-sectionally averaged fluid velocity at location x and time t, and $A(x, t)$ is the cross-sectional area of the vessel at location x and time t.

(b)   Consider now steady flow. What can you conclude about the relationship between $u(x, t)$ and $A(x, t)$?

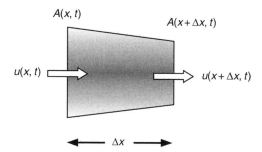

3 Steady and unsteady Bernoulli equation and momentum conservation

(16 problems)

3.1. An incompressible fluid is pumped at flow rate Q out of a pipe into the center of a very large reservoir. You may assume that the fluid flows radially outward from the end of the pipe in all directions, that the pipe itself does not perturb the flow, and that the flow is steady.

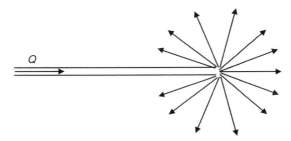

(a) Find the speed of the fluid, $v(r)$, where r is measured outwards from the tip of the pipe.

(b) Assuming inviscid flow, and neglecting gravitational effects, determine the pressure in the reservoir, $p(r)$. Assume that the reservoir pressure far from the end of the pipe is constant and equal to p_0.

3.2. In a simplified model of flow entering the aorta from the left heart, blood passes from a large chamber (the left ventricle, much larger than the aorta) into a long, rigid, straight tube of cross-sectional area A. The flow rate is increasing linearly with time. The pressure at the distal end of the tube is held constant at p_e.

(a) Calculate the pressure in the ventricle on the assumption that the flow is inviscid and quasi-steady (i.e. the temporal acceleration is unimportant).

(b) Evaluate the contribution to the ventricular pressure due to flow acceleration, and determine a criterion as to whether or not the flow can be treated as quasi-steady.

3.3. We are considering the design of a spray painter. Fluid, with a density ρ and a surface tension σ, is ejected from a nozzle, forming an initially continuous stream of constant velocity v_0 and radius R. Then, due to surface tension, the fluid breaks up into a stream of droplets each a distance L_2 from its neighbor. Finally, the stream of droplets is further broken up by a screen into a fine mist of cross-sectional area A_m and bulk (average) density ρ_m. In all of the following, you may neglect any effects due to viscosity.

Note that only part (a) asks for an order-of-magnitude estimate; parts (b) and (c) require exact expressions. You may neglect the role of surface tension in parts (b) and (c) only, not in part (a).

(a)   Obtain an order-of-magnitude estimate, in terms of the parameters given above, of the time τ it takes for the fluid stream to break up into a stream of droplets, assuming that this time is independent of the fluid velocity v_0. (The fluid travels a distance $L_1 = v_0 \tau$ during this time.)

(b)   Determine the time-averaged force acting on the screen. You may ignore the role of surface tension.

(c)   Considering the region upstream of the screen, determine expressions for the velocity of the droplets (v_d) and their radius (R_d) as functions of the given parameters. You may again neglect the role of surface tension.

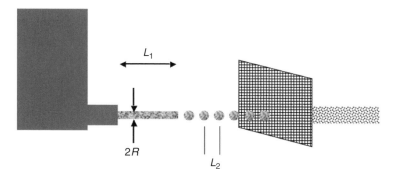

3.4. In an aneurysm, a blood vessel becomes locally dilated. The cause of this dilation is unknown. Here we investigate the hemodynamic consequences of an aneurysm.

Consider the simplified model of an aneurysm shown overleaf. Let the cross-sectional area of the entering and exiting circular blood vessel be A_0 and let that of the aneurysm be A_2. Let the fluid velocity entering be v_0. We wish to find out how the pressure in this vessel is modified by the aneurysm and what tension forces are generated in the vessel wall due to the presence of the aneurysm.

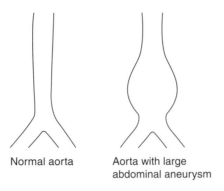

Normal aorta   Aorta with large abdominal aneurysm

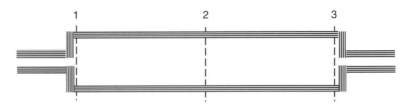

Let the blood be of density ρ. The velocity v_2 can be assumed to be uniform across the cross-section A_2. At location 1, the velocity is zero everywhere except at the area A_0 where the fluid enters the aneurysm at a velocity of v_0. The same is true for the velocity at location 3.

Assume that, at locations 1 and 2, the pressures p_1 and p_2 are uniform across the cross-sectional area. Let p_3 be the pressure in the stream as it exits the aneurysm. Let ρ, A_0, A_2, and v_0 be known. You may ignore viscous shear on the vessel walls.

(a) Find the velocities v_2 and v_3.
(b) Explain where the Bernoulli equation can be applied in this problem and where it cannot. (Hint: where do you expect turbulence to occur?)
(c) Find an expression for $p_1 - p_2$.
(d) Find an expression for $p_1 - p_3$.
(e) Sketch the axial pressure distribution.
(f) Derive an expression for the net axial force F which the vessel wall needs to support because of the aneurysm.

3.5. In atherosclerosis, blood vessels can become progressively obstructed with "plaque," known as an atheroma. These atheromas can rupture, and their contents can flow downstream to block the arterial system at another location. When this occurs in the brain, a stroke often results. We are interested in determining the forces acting on the atheroma (see the figure below). Assume that blood of density ρ is flowing at a steady flow rate through a circular blood vessel that has a cross-sectional area of A. Let the atheroma decrease the area of the vessel to a minimum area of A_2. Assume that, at locations 1, 2, and 3, the respective pressures p_1, p_2, and p_3 are uniform across the cross-sectional area. The velocities v_1 and v_3 are uniform across the cross-section; however, the velocity v_2 is uniform across the area A_2, but zero across the remaining area $(A - A_2)$. Let ρ, A, A_2, and v_1 be known.

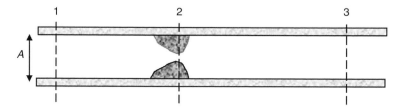

(a) Find the velocities v_2 and v_3 in terms of v_1.
(b) Find an expression for $p_3 - p_2$; you may neglect viscous shear forces along the vessel wall between locations 2 and 3. Note that the distance between A_2 and the edge of the atheroma is short compared with the distance over which p_2 changes to p_3.
(c) Derive an expression for the force F exerted by the fluid on the atheroma. You may assume that the surface of the atheroma leading up to the constriction is relatively smooth, and that the flow is along steady streamlines in this region.

Hint: be careful about where you apply the Bernoulli equation!

3.6. A device used for measuring blood pressure consists of a rigid catheter (of length L and radius R) with a pressure transducer at one end of the line and a needle at the other. The system is entirely filled with saline (of density ρ). The needle is inserted into an artery. For this problem, you can ignore the needle, i.e. assume that the catheter effectively goes directly into the artery. You may assume that the density of any fluid entering the catheter is ρ and that the flow is inviscid. You may also assume that the catheter radius is much smaller than the balloon radius.

The pressure transducer consists of a spherical balloon that stretches when the pressure (P_b) inside the balloon increases. This stretch is measured electronically. The pressure inside the balloon is related to the volume of the balloon by

$$P_b(t) = V_b(t)/C$$

where C is the compliance of the balloon, which is known.

As the blood pressure in the artery, $P_a(t)$, increases, a small amount of fluid enters the catheter, thus increasing the pressure and volume of the balloon.

(a) Find a differential equation for $P_b(t)$ as a function of $P_a(t)$, time (t), and the other given variables in the problem.

(b) What recommendations do you have for designing the system such that the pressure within the transducer will be very similar to that in the artery?

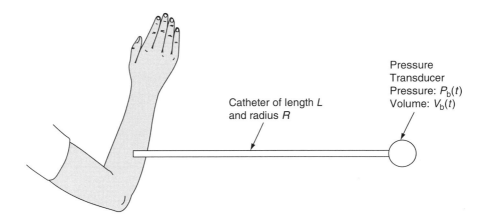

Catheter of length L and radius R

Pressure Transducer
Pressure: $P_b(t)$
Volume: $V_b(t)$

3.7. A squid propels itself by squeezing its body and thereby ejecting a jet of water that propels it forward. It then re-inflates itself with water and repeats the process in order to continue to move along. We consider here an experimental study carried out while the squid is held stationary. All questions below apply to the propulsion phase of motion.

Consider a model of this process wherein the squid is considered to be a cylinder of uniform radius at any point in time, $R(t)$ (as shown in the right figure); $R(t=0) = R_0$. Let water have a density of ρ, and assume the process to be inviscid.

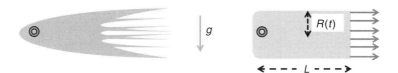

g $R(t)$ L

(a) If $dR(t)/dt = -\gamma$, a constant, during the propulsion cycle, find $V_{\text{exit}}(t)$, the velocity of the fluid exiting the back of the squid.

(b) Let the front of the squid be located at $x = 0$, and let the back of the squid be located at $x = L$. Find the maximum pressure inside the squid, relative to the pressure in the water surrounding the squid, P_0. You may ignore hydrostatic changes in pressure.

(c) How much force $F(t)$ would have to be applied to the squid in order to keep it stationary?

3.8. Consider an inviscid flow in which fluid is pushed by a piston of cross-sectional area A_0 through a nozzle. The nozzle has a short section of constant area A_0 and length L_0, followed by a section where the area decreases exponentially according to

$$A(x) = A_0 \exp(-2x/L) \quad \text{for } 0 \le x \le L$$

In this nozzle L_0, the section upstream of $x = 0$, is much shorter than L: $L_0 \ll L$.

Initially, the fluid is everywhere stationary. Then, at $t = 0$, the piston begins to push with a constant force F (the piston moves without friction through the nozzle and has negligible mass). We are interested in modeling the process before the piston reaches $x = 0$.

(a) Find a differential equation that describes $v_1(t)$, the velocity of the fluid exiting the nozzle, in terms of known quantities given in the problem statement above.
(b) After a little while, $v_1(t)$ approaches a steady-state velocity (the piston not yet having reached $x = 0$). What is the steady-state velocity of the fluid exiting the nozzle?
(c) When $v_1(t)$ reaches a steady state, what is the restraining force in the strut that keeps the nozzle from moving in the axial direction?

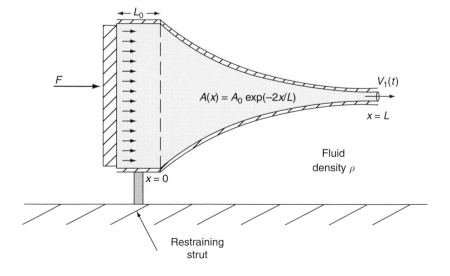

3.9. A heart replacement needs to be attached to the aorta. We are interested in determining the force, F, that must be supported by the sutures attaching the heart replacement to the aorta.

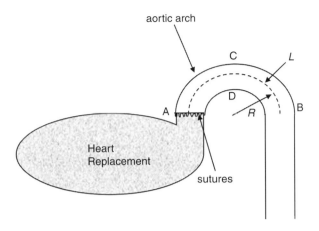

Shown in the figure is the aortic arch as attached to the artificial heart. The flow rate being delivered to the aorta is $Q(t) = Q_0[1 - \cos(\omega t)]$, while the pressure supplied at the root of the aorta is $P(t) = P_0[1 - \cos(\omega t)]$. The frequency ω is in units of radians per second. The blood has a density of ρ. The aorta has a diameter of d, and this can be assumed to be constant along the length of the aortic arch. It has a radius of curvature of R, and its length in the streamwise direction from A to B is L $(L \gg d)$.

You may ignore the effects of gravity. The flow can be considered to be inviscid.

(a) Find the vertical force, $F(t)$, that must be supported by the sutures of the aorta to the heart replacement at A. You may assume that there is no force within the wall of the aorta at point B. For this part only, you may also assume that the velocity of the blood is uniform across any cross-section, and thus you may ignore the effects of streamline curvature.

(b) Very roughly estimate the difference in fluid pressure between points C and D in the aortic arch.

3.10. A venous graft is to be sewn onto an artery to replace a damaged vessel. We want to evaluate what forces the sutures which are holding the vessels together might need to support.

The blood has density ρ. Assume the flow is inviscid. You may also assume that there are no axial stresses in the wall of the blood vessel at its downstream end (other than those generated by atmospheric pressure). All solutions must be in terms of given quantities. The pressure in the wall of the blood vessel and the surrounding tissue can be take to be P_{atm}.

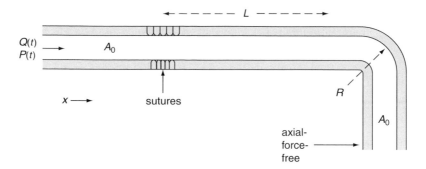

(a) Let $Q(t) = Q_0[1 + \cos(\omega t + \delta)]$ and let the pressure upstream of the suture be $P(t) = P_0[1 + \sin(\omega t)] + P_{atm}$; δ is the phase angle between the flow and pressure. Downstream of the sutures, the vessel is straight for a distance L before undergoing a tight $90°$ turn with radius of curvature R ($R \ll L$). The cross-sectional area of the vessel is constant and equal to A_0. Estimate the axial force on the sutures as a function of given quantities.

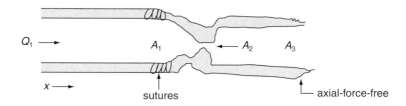

Now, consider the effects of a constriction in the flow downstream of the suture as might occur due to the development of a plaque in the vessel wall. Let this plaque reduce the vessel lumen area from A_1 to A_2 as shown in the figure. Downstream of the constriction the vessel opens to an area A_3, with $A_3 < A_1$. Let the flow and pressure be steady, with $Q = Q_1$ (constant), and let the pressure upstream of the suture be $P_1 + P_{atm}$ (constant).

(b) Determine the pressure downstream of the constriction at the location labeled as A_3 where the flow is uniform.

(c) Roughly estimate the force acting on the sutures (assuming there are smooth streamlines upstream of the point of maximum constriction).

3.11. There are many bifurcations in the flow pathways of the body. At each bifurcation, the flow streamlines must curve, and thus it is important to understand the influence of this curvature on the flow. Consider a straight rectangular channel of height h and width W with a flow rate Q passing through the channel. Let the velocity in this straight section be uniform across the channel, and let the density of the fluid be ρ.

Now let the flow enter a part of the channel that is gently curving, with a radius of curvature R ($h \ll R$) (see the figure). You may ignore gravity and viscosity.

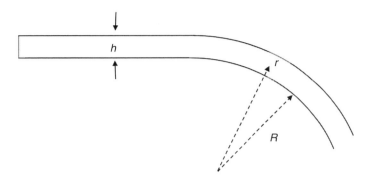

(a) Does $P(r)$ change with r and, if so, does it increase or decrease with increasing r? Make a guess at a velocity distribution, $v(r)$.

(b) Find $v(r)$.

3.12. A soap bubble (surface tension σ) is attached to a very narrow glass tube as shown in the figure. The initial radius of the bubble is R_0. The pressure inside the bubble is greater than atmospheric pressure due to surface tension. At $t = 0$, the end of the glass tube is abruptly opened. In this problem, we will only consider times (t) such that the bubble radius $R(t)$ (which is unknown) is <u>much</u> larger than

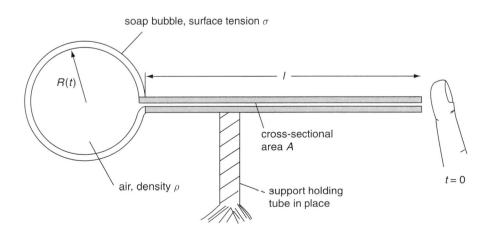

the radius of the glass tube. The flow can be considered to be inviscid and incompressible, and gravitational effects can be neglected. All answers should be in terms of ρ (air density), σ, A, l, t, and R_0 (not all of these variables will need to be used).

(a) First consider the "quasi-steady" emptying of the bubble such that the unsteady velocity term in Euler's or Bernoulli's equation ($\partial V/\partial t$) can be neglected. Find the rate of change of pressure inside the bubble as a function of time: $dP(t)/dt$.

(b) For the same quasi-steady conditions, find the force (F) necessary in order to hold the glass tube in place.

(c) Now consider the instant when the glass tube is <u>first</u> opened. Find dV_{exit}/dt at $t = 0$, where V_{exit} is the air velocity flowing out of the glass tube [1].

3.13. Engineers for a company selling medical products have developed an inexpensive, hand-held device for monitoring peak expiratory flow rates in asthmatics. The device, shown in the figure, consists of a rigid cylinder (of diameter D) with a long, narrow slit down the side (of width $h \ll D$) and a close-fitting, spring-loaded piston diaphragm. Expired air enters the chamber of the peak-flow meter from the left through the mouthpiece, then exits via the slit *at a uniform velocity* and at an angle α to the vertical direction. The length of the slit available for flow, x, is equal to the displacement of the piston. Gas exits from the slit in the form of a jet into the atmosphere at pressure p_a.

Assume that the flow is steady *and inviscid*, that the piston moves without friction, and that the displacement is linearly proportional to the force f acting on it:

$$f = kx$$

Determine x as a function of α, Q, h, D, k, ρ, and p_a.

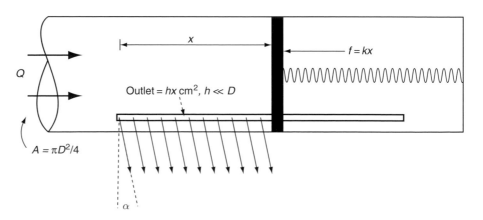

3.14. Blood flow in smaller arteries (but not in the capillaries or arterioles, where the size of a red blood cell is comparable to the vessel diameter) has a nearly Poiseuille velocity profile:

$$v(r) = v_{\max}\left[1 - \left(\frac{r}{R}\right)^2\right]$$

This velocity profile is caused by viscous forces that also cause the pressure of the fluid to drop along the length of the blood vessel. The relationship between the pressure gradient (dP/dx) and flow (Q) in that vessel (for steady, fully developed flow) is given as

$$\frac{dp}{dx} = -\frac{8\mu Q}{\pi R^4}$$

where x is the length along the blood vessel, μ is the fluid viscosity, and R is the radius of the blood vessel.

Consider a small artery that branches at an angle of 30° as shown below (each branch 15° from the horizontal). The radius of the artery (R_a) is twice that of the identical daughter branches, and the length of the daughter branches is the same as that of the upstream artery (L).

Let the flow rate passing through the large blood vessel be Q. Determine how much the horizontal force on these vessels would change if the top daughter branch became blocked at its end. You may ignore the effect of the shear forces on the vessel walls.

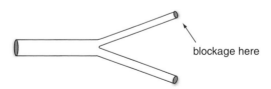

blockage here

3.15. A monolayer of cells is kept moist by a stream of saline (shaded in the figure) that is continuously dropped on to these cells. We are interested in making sure that this stream does not injure the cells beneath it. The saline (density ρ) flows at volumetric flow rate Q out of a spout of radius R_0 and lands on a layer (thickness L) of saline that overlies the cells. The dropped saline mixes turbulently with the saline overlying the cells. You may ignore the effects of surface tension for this problem.

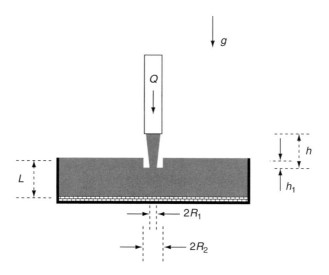

(a) The shape of the falling stream is approximately that of a cone (volume V_0). Find the radius of the stream (R_1) as it hits the layer of fluid on top of the cells in terms of the given quantities and the height h shown on the figure.

(b) This stream will depress the saline layer on top of the cells in the region where it strikes. We want to make sure that that saline layer does not become so depressed that the cells are exposed to the direct force of the falling saline. You may assume that the radius of this depressed region is R_2, which is only very slightly larger than the radius of the incoming saline stream, R_1. Find the depth (h_1) by which the surface will be depressed by the incoming stream.

Note the following points.

(i) The fluid leaves the system by very slowly overflowing at the edges of the container.

(ii) Viscous effects can be neglected.

(iii) While the shape of the depression is shown with a sharp border, in reality surface tension would smooth this out. This can be neglected in your calculation.

3.16. The goal here is to derive the equation for one-dimensional wave propagation in a blood vessel, which describes how a disturbance in pressure or vessel cross-sectional area at one location propagates along the vessel.

(a) Consider the mass-conservation law for flow through a compliant vessel such as that found in Problem 2.11. Now let the area of the tube be related to the internal pressure at any location by $A(x) = A_0 + [\alpha(P(x) - P_{ext}]$, where A_0 is the

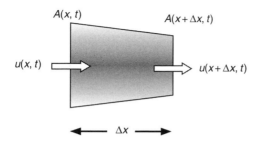

undeformed area of the tube and P_{ext} is the pressure surrounding the vessel. Find a relationship between the pressure in the vessel and the velocity.

(b) A second relationship between the pressure in the vessel and the velocity can be found from the one-dimensional unsteady Bernoulli equation. Assuming that the fluid velocity is very small, combine these two equations to find a single partial differential equation that describes the pressure as a function of space and time. This equation is called the wave equation. (Hint: small velocity means that variations in other parameters will be small also.)

(c) Solve this equation assuming that $P(x) = f(x - ct)$, where f is a smooth but otherwise arbitrary function. Show that c is the wave speed, and determine this speed in terms of parameters given in the problem.

4 Viscous flow

(33 problems)

4.1. When blood is taken out of the body for processing into an extracorporeal device, a major concern is that the level of shear stress to which the blood is exposed should be less than a critical level (roughly 1000 dyne/cm²). For exposure to shear-stress levels higher than this, lysis of the red blood cells can occur, together with platelet activation and initiation of the clotting process.

Consider the flow of blood through a device that has a set of parallel tubes each with a diameter of 1 mm and a length of 10 cm. What is the maximum pressure drop that should be used for such a device if the highest shear levels in the device occur in these tubes? (Blood has a viscosity about five times that of water.) You may neglect entry effects and treat the flow as fully developed.

4.2. A parallel-plate flow chamber is to be designed to study the effects of shear stress on adhesion of leukocytes to endothelia. However, endothelial cells can be damaged by shear stress greater than 400 dyne/cm². The width of the flow channel is to be 1 cm and its length 5 cm. The flow is to be driven by gravity, and a fluid column 1 m in height is available. The system must work both for saline and for blood. What should be the maximum separation ($s \ll 1$ cm) between the two plates such that the endothelial cells are not damaged? The schematic diagram below is not to scale. You may neglect entry effects and treat the flow as fully developed.

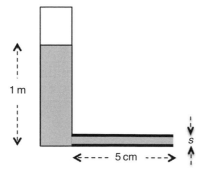

4.3. A dialysis unit is being designed. It will consist of a large number of small hollow fibers arranged in parallel. Blood will flow inside the fibers, each of which is 30 cm long. It is desired that the hold-up volume (the volume of blood needed to fill all the fibers) should be no more than 80 ml, and that the total pressure drop across the fibers should be no more than 10^5 dyne/cm^2 at a total flow rate of 50 ml/s. If the blood viscosity is 3.5 cP and the density of the blood is 1.05 g/cm^3, how many fibers should be used, and of what diameter should they be, so as to meet the design conditions? (Hint: before you start this problem, think about what kind of flow you will have in these fibers.) Justify any assumption you make.

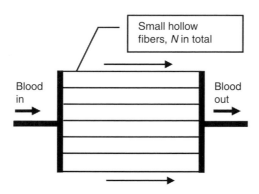

4.4. The shear stress level in arteries is regulated such that, when a higher (or lower) shear level is sensed by the endothelium of an artery, the artery alters its radius so that the shear level returns to its optimal value. This optimal value, τ_0, is relatively constant throughout the arterial tree. On the basis of this criterion, determine how the flow rate depends on the artery diameter in such an arterial tree. You may assume steady flow conditions.

4.5. Two very large plates (of area A) are separated by a thin fluid-filled gap of height h. A force F is applied to the upper plate and the resulting upper-plate velocity V_p is measured. These quantities allow the effective viscosity (μ_{eff}) of the fluid in the gap to be calculated as

$$\mu_{eff} = \frac{F/A}{V/h}$$

When the gap is filled with blood, a plasma-skimming layer of thickness Δ occurs at both plates. You may treat the core fluid and each plasma-skimming layer as Newtonian, with viscosities of μ_c and μ_p, respectively.

For blood, what is μ_{eff} in terms of μ_c, μ_p, Δ, and h?

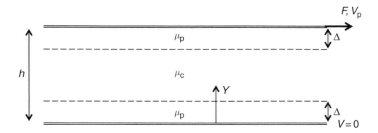

4.6. Optical traps (or "tweezers") can capture cells and hold them in place. We would like to determine how much force such a set of tweezers can apply. Using microparticles (of radius 2 μm) and a microscope, describe how you might do an experiment to determine this force for an optical trap in your laboratory.

4.7. Laser light can be used to create an optical trap that holds particles in position. In this application, laser light is used to hold a cell in the middle of a flow field while assaying the effect of the flow on the cell using fluorescence-based imaging techniques.

Consider the flow in a cylindrical tube (of radius $R = 0.1$ mm and length $L = 10$ cm) as shown below (the diagram is not to scale). The cell is to be trapped in the middle of the tube ($r = 0$, $x = 5$ cm). The cell has a radius of $a = 5$ μm and a density of 1.1 g/cm^3. The cell is small enough that it does not influence the flow through the tube.

The pressure drop (ΔP) available to drive flow through the tube can be set as low as 1000 g/cm per s^2. The perfusion fluid, saline, has a viscosity of 0.01 g/cm per s and a density of 1 g/cm^3. If the laser can generate a force of 250 pN (250 × 10^{-12} N), determine whether the cell can be held stationary by the laser in this experiment.

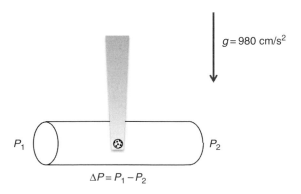

4.8. The airways of the lung are coated with a thin liquid lining of highly viscous fluid (of viscosity μ and density ρ). The thickness of this liquid lining (h) is much less than the radius of these airways (R). In the larger airways, cilia on the airway wall beat up and down, "pumping" the fluid upward (toward the mouth) and opposing the pull of gravity. We can model this process by assuming that the velocity of the fluid at the airway wall ($y = 0$) is given as V_0 (see the figure).

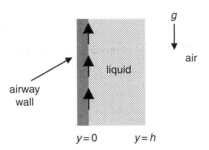

(a)   Draw the velocity profile $V(y)$ of the fluid flow in the liquid lining.
(b)   Solve for this velocity profile.
(c)   What value must V_0 have in order for the net volume flow rate of this liquid to be upward?

4.9. One method used to test the adhesion strength of a cell population is a radial flow assay. Cell culture medium enters the system at the center of a disk-shaped chamber in which cells are adhering to the bottom surface. As the flow moves radially outward from the center, the flow speed, and therefore the shear force exerted on each cell, decreases. The cells closest to the center experience the highest levels of force and are torn loose from the substrate. Beyond some critical radial distance, r_c, the adhesion strength is sufficient that the cells remain attached. Here we consider both the flow of the medium and the effect it has on the individual cells. (Note that the cells in the drawing are shown much larger than actual size.) For parts (a)–(d) below, you may assume viscous-dominated flow.

(a)   Obtain an expression for the mean speed of the fluid as a function of Q, the volume flow rate entering the chamber, r, the distance measured from the axis, and h, the height of the flow region.
(b)   Sketch (and calculate) the velocity profile inside the gap, namely $v_r = v_r(z)$, where z is measured vertically upward from the cell surface (at a position $r \gg h$).
(c)   Obtain an expression for the shear stress acting on the cell that shows the dependence of the shear stress on the viscosity of the medium (μ), the volume flow rate (Q), the radial distance (r), and the channel height (h).

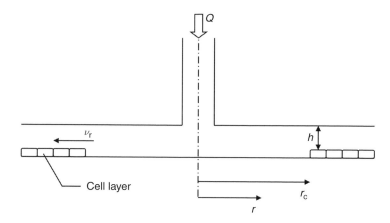

(d) Using a force balance on a single cell (of surface area A), obtain an *approximate* (scaling) expression for the maximum adhesion strength f (force per unit area), in terms of given parameters.

(e) Give a quantitative criterion in terms of given quantities that would allow you to evaluate whether or not the assumption of viscous-dominated flow is justified.

4.10. Under normal conditions, the lateral surfaces of epithelial cells in the lung are separated by a small distance, making a space referred to as the lateral intercellular space (LIS). When smooth muscle in the walls of an airway constricts, the cells are pushed together, squeezing the fluid within the LIS out through the bottom (tight junctions near the top (apical) surface of the cells prevent outflow from the top).

Assume that the lateral cell membranes can be treated as two flat surfaces that remain flat and parallel as the distance separating them, h, is reduced at a rate dh/dt, and that the flow is viscous-dominated. Each of the following is given: h, dh/dt, the length of the LIS, L, and the fluid viscosity, μ.

(a) Obtain an expression for the flow rate per unit depth (into the paper) as a function of the distance, x, from the top of the LIS.

(b) Obtain an expression for the velocity profile, $v_x(y)$, assuming the flow to be "fully developed" (i.e. locally Poiseuille), in terms of the pressure gradient, dp/dx, and the other parameters of the problem.

(c) Using your result from (b), obtain an expression for the maximum pressure inside the LIS. Where does this maximum occur? (Let the pressure at $x = L$ be P_{tissue}.)

(d) Give a quantitative criterion in terms of given quantities that would allow you to evaluate whether or not the assumption of viscous flow is justified.

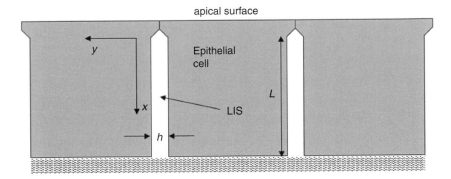

apical surface

4.11. When blood flows through small blood vessels (vessels of diameter less than 300 μm), it behaves somewhat strangely due to the red blood cells (RBCs). Because of their size, they cannot be immediately adjacent to the vessel wall; furthermore, lift forces also move them away from the wall. Owing to these phenomena, the fluid behaves as if it had two phases: the thin layer next to the wall, known as the plasma-skimming layer, which is nearly pure plasma with a viscosity of $\mu_s = 0.013$ g/cm per s; and the whole blood in the rest of the capillary, with a viscosity of $\mu_b = 0.04$ g/cm per s. The two layers have the same density, $\rho = 1$ g/ml.

We are interested in modeling the flow of blood through a microfluidic device that is used in a biotechnology application. In particular, we want to make sure that the shear stress experienced by the RBCs does not exceed τ_{max}.

Blood flows through channels that have a height of $h = 80$ μm, a width of $w = 2$ mm, and a length of 1 cm. Let the thickness of the plasma-only region near each wall be $t = 10$ μm.

(a) Find the maximum pressure drop (ΔP) that can be used to drive this flow such that the shear stress will not exceed τ_{max} for any RBC. You may assume that the plasma and blood layers do not mix.

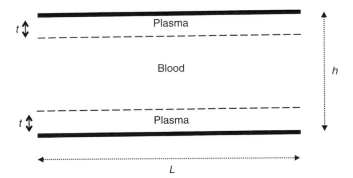

(b) Find the maximum velocity of the plasma (not blood) passing through the channel at this pressure drop.

4.12. The airways in the lung are covered with a thin liquid lining. Gravity acts to pull this fluid down into the lung, while cilia in the upper airways pump this fluid upward. However, in the lower airways, there are few cilia and surface tension becomes more important in this balance. During a cough, air motion can be important.

Assume an airway diameter of 2 mm and a fluid lining of 10 μm (thin enough that the curvature of the liquid lining can be neglected in this problem). Ignoring effects of cilia and surface tension, what flow rate of air is necessary to cause <u>all of the fluid</u> in the liquid lining of this airway to move upward during a cough? The viscosity of the liquid lining is 0.01 g/cm per s and its density is 1 g/ml; the viscosity of the air is 1.9×10^{-4} g/cm per s. Assume steady-state conditions.

When considering the boundary condition at the interface between the moving air and the airway liquid, recall that the flow of air is affecting the flow of liquid.

4.13. The tear film (of density 1 g/cm^3 and viscosity 0.013 g/cm per s) bathes the cornea and protects it from drying out. Treat the cornea as a vertical planar surface, and assume that the tear film has a uniform thickness of $h = 5$ μm. Let the length of the cornea (in the flow-wise direction) be 1 cm.

Assume that a blink occurs every 5 s (which replenishes the fluid layer on the surface of the cornea).

(a) Find what fraction of the tear film is lost between blinks (assume steady flow between blinks).
(b) The surface of the tear film has proteins that alter the surface tension. Owing to their presence, a Marangoni force can develop. This force can be modeled by assuming that the surface of the tear film become immobile. How would this alter your answer to part (a)?

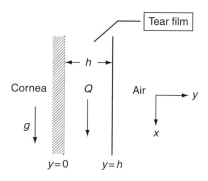

4.14. Flow through connective tissues in the body, such as cartilage, the renal glomerulus, and the interstitium, occurs through complicated flow passages that are difficult to characterize. One approach is to treat these tissues as *porous media*, and to apply Darcy's law, which relates the pressure drop (ΔP) across a porous medium to its *permeability* (K):

$$\Delta P = \frac{\mu Q L}{K A}$$

where μ is the fluid viscosity, Q is the flow rate, L is the length of the porous medium in the flow-wise direction, and A is the cross-sectional area of the medium (solid plus void) facing the flow.

A simple model of a porous medium is to treat it as a number of long tortuous pores that pass through the medium. Let the medium be characterized as having n pores per unit cross-sectional area. Let the pores have an average radius of a, and an average length of τL, where τ is the *tortuosity* of the pore path. (You may ignore all inertial effects.)

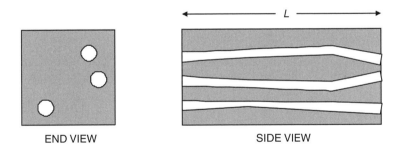

END VIEW   SIDE VIEW

(a) Find the porosity (the void volume per total volume) and the specific surface area (the surface area of the pore walls per unit volume) of this medium as functions of n, a, and τ ONLY.

(b) Find the permeability as a function of the porosity, the specific surface, and the tortuosity of the medium ONLY. This relationship is known as the Carman–Kozeny equation.

(c) Typical extracellular matrices in the body have a permeability of 2×10^{-14} cm^2 and a porosity of 80% (or higher). Calculate a typical pore diameter of such a medium. Assume a tortuosity of 1.5.

Note that the Carman–Kozeny equation becomes less accurate as the porosity increases. See the next problem for a better treatment of this situation for high-porosity media.

4.15. As stated in the previous problem, flow through connective tissues in the body, such as cartilage, the renal glomerulus, and the interstitium, occurs through complicated flow passages that are difficult to characterize. One approach is to treat these tissues as *porous media*, and to apply Darcy's law, which relates the pressure drop (ΔP) across a porous medium to its *permeability* (K):

$$\Delta P = \frac{\mu Q L}{KA}$$

where μ is the fluid viscosity, Q is the flow rate, L is the length of the porous medium in the flow-wise direction, and A is the cross-sectional area facing the flow. Here K is an intrinsic property that does not depend on the dimensions of the medium (L or A), and depends only on the structure of the medium at the microscale.

We previously considered a model of a porous medium that treated it as a number of long tortuous pores that pass through the medium. However, such an approach is useful only if the porosity of the medium is less than 80% or so. Most biological porous media have very high porosities, and flow through them is better described as flow over objects rather than flow through tubes.

Assume that a porous medium can be described as a set of objects, each of which generates a drag force of $F = c\mu UR$, where c is a constant (6π for a sphere), μ is the viscosity of the fluid, U is the average velocity of the fluid passing over each object, and R is the radius (or another characteristic dimension) of the object facing the flow. Let n be the number of objects per unit volume.

(a) Find K for such a porous medium.
(b) State the limitations on Q/A for which your answer to part (a) is valid.
(c) Now let Q be much higher than the limitation found in part (b). Roughly estimate F and K for such a porous medium. (Hint: use dimensional analysis.)

4.16. A cell-separation (fractionation) system is based on cell density. Cells are injected at the center of a tube of radius R, and are carried by fluid flowing at flow rate Q. Dense cells fall quickly under the action of gravity, adhere to the tube wall, and hence do not pass out of the tube. Assume that the concentration of cells is low enough that the laminar flow in the tube is not perturbed by the presence of the cells.

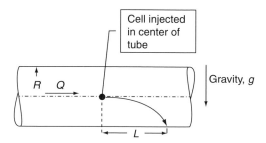

Let the cells be spherical, with radius a, and let them have a density of $\rho + \Delta\rho$, where ρ is the density of the flowing fluid.

Find the axial distance (L) that a cell travels before it hits the bottom wall. You need to use the fact that, in fully developed flow in the presence of gravity, the pressure distribution in the vertical direction is hydrostatic and the axial velocity profile is the familiar parabolic shape. You may assume that the cell is spherical, that it reaches its terminal (falling) velocity nearly immediately after injection into the tube, and that it gets carried axially at the local fluid velocity in the tube. State any other assumptions you make.

4.17. At very large values of hematocrit, red blood cells (RBCs) interact with one another strongly. One model of such an interaction is shown in the figure below, in which RBCs form "lines" separated by gaps. (This is an appropriate model for high-shear flow in a planar channel.) Assume that the RBCs pack together in each "line" so that the space between cells in a given "line" can be neglected. For a hematocrit of $H = 0.75$, calculate μ_{eff} in such a system in a Couette-flow apparatus as shown below. Assume that all RBCs have the same thickness (w), that RBCs have the shape shown below, that all fluid gaps between lines have uniform thickness (t), and that the plasma viscosity is 1 cP. You may consider the flow to be two-dimensional. State other assumptions. (Note that the RBCs in the figure are not to scale. In a real channel there would be many such RBC "lines". See [2].)

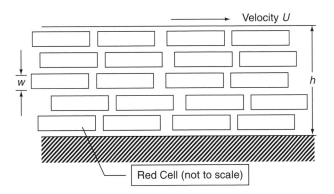

Red Cell (not to scale)

4.18. In the lung, some particles are removed by inertial impact with the walls as they pass through the airways. Specifically, since their density is higher than that of the air carrying them, they do not exactly track the fluid path when the path is curved.

Consider one such curved vessel downstream from a bifurcation (see the figure below). For simplicity, allow the flow passage to be a two-dimensional channel of width W instead of a round tube, and further allow that the air everywhere be moving uniformly with a velocity of V in the direction of flow. Let the radius of curvature be $R \gg W$. Assume that air of density ρ_a and viscosity μ enters this airway uniformly loaded with aerosol particles of radius $s \ll R$ and density ρ. Calculate what fraction of the particles will intercept the wall and be removed from the flow as it leaves this section of the airways. You can ignore gravity. The total turning angle of the bend is 90°.

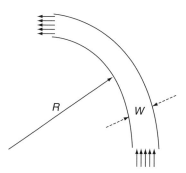

4.19. Consider a very long (length L) hollow cylinder of radius R placed in a very large body of water that can be assumed to be infinite in size for the purposes of this problem. The cylinder walls are much, much thinner than its radius. The cylinder is rotated at a constant angular velocity of Ω about its long axis (centerline). You may neglect gravity.

(a)   Find the velocity of the fluid, $v(r)$, of the fluid inside and outside of the tube, where r is the radial distance from the center of the tube.
(b)   Find the externally applied torque per unit cylinder length necessary to keep the cylinder turning at the constant angular velocity Ω.
(c)   Now suppose that the tube continues to rotate while an axial flow (with flow rate Q) enters at $x = 0$ and leaves at $x = L$, where x is the axial position in the tube. Assume a bubble of radius $a_0 \ll R$ enters the tube with this flow at $r = 0.1R$. What is the radial location of this bubble when it leaves the tube? (You may assume that the axial flow is very slow, so Coriolis forces may be neglected, i.e. the net flow is the superposition of the axial flow and that computed in part (a).)

4.20. Consider a capillary completely filled with red blood cells (RBCs) as shown in the figure. We wish to derive an expression for the effective viscosity of the RBC suspension passing through this capillary compared with that of plasma (of viscosity μ_p) alone passing through this capillary. You may assume that the small amount of fluid between two adjacent RBCs moves at the same velocity as that of the RBCs.

(a) Let the velocity of each RBC be given as v, and let the average pressure gradient $(-dP/dx)$ driving the flow be G. Find the velocity profile of the fluid in the gap $(0 < y < 2h)$ between each RBC and the capillary wall. You may assume for all parts of this problem that $2h \ll R$.

(b) Now do a force balance on the column of RBCs and find the velocity v as a function of G.

(c) Find the effective viscosity of the RBC suspension passing through this capillary as a function of plasma viscosity and other relevant parameters. The effective viscosity is that viscosity which you would measure if you assumed the fluid to exhibit Newtonian behavior.

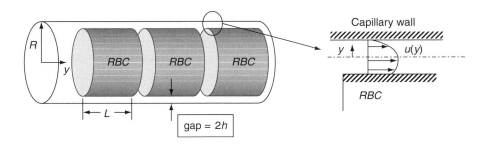

4.21. Red blood cells (RBCs) have a biconcave shape. Hydrodynamically they can be described as cylindrical disks that have a diameter of approximately $d = 7.6\ \mu m$ and a thickness of $l = 2.8\ \mu m$. Capillary diameters are just a little smaller than the diameter of the RBCs, thus the RBCs "squeeze" through these vessels. Actually, there is a thin lubricating layer between the RBC and the capillary wall, of thickness approximately $h = 0.1\ \mu m$, through which the plasma flows around the RBC.

We want to determine the pressure drop through a section of the capillary with one RBC in it. Assume that the RBC moves at an average speed of $v_{RBC} = 0.05$ cm/s.

(a) Roughly estimate the shear forces acting to slow down the RBC.

(b) From this estimate, determine the pressure drop across the RBC.

(c) Use your answer to part (b) to justify any assumption you needed to make for part (a).

(d) If the distance between RBCs is L, estimate the total axial pressure drop from one RBC to the corresponding location on the adjacent RBC.

(e) Sketch the velocity profile of the plasma near the RBC to compare with that for the plasma far away.

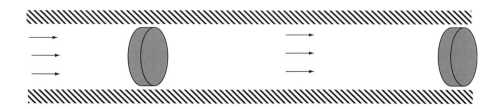

4.22. In your eye, between the iris (the brown or blue part of your eye) and the cornea (the front part of your eye) there is a clear fluid known as aqueous humor. The iris is at a temperature of 37 °C, while the cornea is cooler, being at a temperature of approximately 33 °C. The temperature difference causes the density of aqueous humor right next to the iris to be slightly lower than that of the aqueous humor next to the cornea, leading to flow known as natural convection. The aqueous humor next to the iris rises, while the aqueous humor next to the cornea falls. Gravity points in the negative y-direction. We wish to model this process.

Let the temperature of the aqueous humor vary linearly between the iris and the cornea, let the density of the aqueous humor in the eye vary with temperature as

$$\rho = (1\,\text{g/cm}^3)[1 - 3.6 \times 10^{-4}\,°\text{C}^{-1}(T - 35\,°\text{C})]$$

and let the viscosity of the aqueous humor be the same as water.

(a) Draw the vertical velocity profile in the aqueous humor.
(b) What do you expect dP/dx to be?
(c) Solve for the pressure gradient (dP/dy) at $x = 0$.
(d) Find the peak velocity in the aqueous humor.

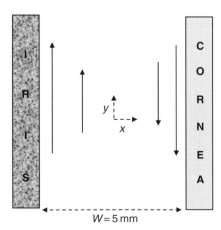

4.23. An apparatus has been built for testing the effect of various drugs on the rate at which an epithelium can pump fluid from its luminal side (the side facing the fluid) to its basal side (which lies on the channel wall). The cells line the top and bottom surface of a flow channel that has a width of h (from top plate to bottom plate; we ignore the thickness of cells), a length L, and a depth into the page of W. Each of these walls is porous so that any fluid pumped by the cells can leave the channel. Let each cell layer pump fluid at a rate of q per unit area of the channel walls (for a total rate of fluid pumped by the cells on the top surface of the channel of S, we have $q = S/A$, where $A = LW$; q has units of length/time). The height of the channel is much less than its length ($h \ll L$).

Fluid enters the channel at the left at a flow rate of Q_0 and a gauge pressure of P_0. Because of the pumping of the cells, the flow rate through the channel decreases as a function of x, the distance from the beginning of the channel. To determine the rate at which the cells are pumping fluid out of the channel, the channel is instrumented with pressure transducers that can measure $P(x)$. We would like to use this information to find the rate at which the cells pump fluid.

The fluid in the channel has a density of ρ and a viscosity of μ. The flow is dominated by viscous effects and is steady.

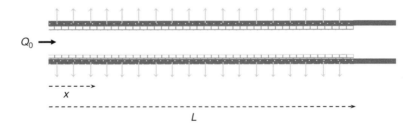

(a) Find the pressure distribution, $P(x)$, in the flow channel if $q = 0$.
(b) Now find the pressure distribution $P(x)$ in the channel for $q \neq 0$.
(c) Given that $P(x = L) = P_e$, find q.
(d) Find the criterion necessary for the assumption that viscous flow dominates to be valid.

All answers must be given in terms of the known quantities given in the problem: x, L, W, h, Q_0, P_0, P_e, ρ, and μ (not all of these parameters need necessarily be used).

4.24. A catheter is used for drug delivery to a tissue. It is a round needle with tiny pores in its surface such that the hydraulic conductivity (flow rate per unit area divided by the pressure drop) of the wall of the needle (see the figure) is $L_p = 1 \times 10^{-5}$ cm^2 s/g. The lumen of the needle is 100 μm in radius. The needle is 2 cm long.

The end of the needle is blocked off, so flow can exit only through the porous walls of the needle. The drug solution to be delivered to the tissue has a viscosity of 0.01 g/cm per s.

(a) If the upstream pressure driving the drug solution into the needle is 5 mm Hg (6.67×10^3 g/cm per s^2), find how many seconds it will take for this catheter to deliver 100 μl of drug to the tissue. You may assume that the tissue is everywhere at atmospheric pressure (0 mm Hg gauge pressure), and that it has negligible transport resistance. The porous section of the needle is sufficiently long that the pressure inside the lumen of the needle at the end of the needle ($z = 2$ cm) is essentially the tissue pressure; in other words, for this part of the problem, the needle can be considered to be essentially infinitely long. Assume locally Poiseuille flow.

(b) Evaluate the assumption that the needle is infinitely long. How much error does this introduce into your answer to part (a)?

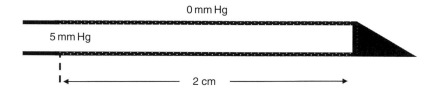

4.25. Consider steady flow of blood (treated as a Newtonian fluid with density ρ and viscosity μ) through an artery (ignore the pulsatile effects). The radius of the blood vessel is determined by the pressure inside the blood vessel, the pressure outside the vessel, and the properties of the vessel wall. Consider an artery whose radius behaves as follows:

$$R = R_0 + \alpha(P - P_{\text{tissue}})$$

where R_0 is the radius of the vessel when the pressure inside the vessel is the same as the tissue pressure.

We are interested in whether the blood vessel will change size appreciably as blood flows through the vessel due to pressure changes in the flowing fluid.

(a) If the tapering of the tube is not too severe, then the flow is "nearly" Poiseuille (dP/dx is not constant, but we can still use the Poiseuille relationship locally). Using an order-of-magnitude analysis of the Navier–Stokes equation, determine a criterion that indicates whether the flow will have a Poiseuille velocity profile.

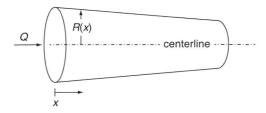

(b) Assuming that this criterion is satisfied, find the pressure drop in a tube of length L, if the inlet pressure is P_1.

(c) Let blood (effective Newtonian viscosity 3.5 cP and density 1.05 g/cm^3) flow through a blood vessel with $\alpha = 5 \times 10^{-7}$ cm^3/dyne and $R_0 = 1$ mm. If Q is 200 ml/min, the average inlet pressure is 70 mm Hg, and we let the tissue pressure be atmospheric, determine the tube radius 4 mm from the inlet.

4.26. As a means of obtaining an estimate for the viscosity of the cytoplasm of a cell in the region of a lamellipod, a flat probe is slowly pushed against the cell surface with constant force, F, while monitoring the probe's displacement (which is quasi-steady). The diameter of the circular probe is d, which is much greater than the local thickness of the cell (h) but much smaller than the overall cell dimension.

(a) Find an expression for the mean radial (horizontal) velocity of the cytoplasm, $v_r(r, t)$ as a function of the rate at which the probe is being lowered, dh/dt, the instantaneous value of h, and the fluid properties.

(b) Noting that the force applied to the probe is balanced by the pressure generated in the cytoplasm beneath it due to the radial flow of the viscous cytoplasm, find the viscosity, μ, of the cytoplasm in terms of the parameters specified. You may assume the flow to be viscous-dominated. You may

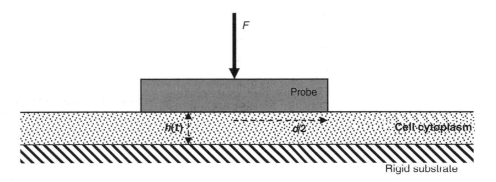

consider the effects of the cell membrane and cytoskeleton to be negligible for the purpose of this analysis.

4.27. Consider a flow between two porous rotating cylinders (length L), the inner cylinder rotating at an angular velocity of ω_1 while the outer cylinder rotates at an angular velocity of ω_2 with $\omega_2 = \omega_1 R_1^2 / R_2^2$. There is also a small radial outward flow of Q. The fluid density is ρ.

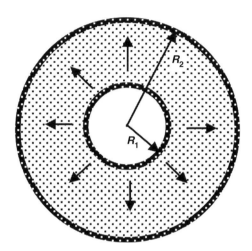

(a) Find the theta direction velocity field $V_\theta(r)$ for $R_1 < r < R_2$.
(b) This device is designed as a bubble trap with fluid entering at R_1 and leaving at R_2. Consider a spherical bubble of radius $a \ll R_1$ that enters with the flow at R_1. What is the minimum value of ω_1 needed in order to ensure that the bubble does not leave with the flow at R_2?

4.28. A rod of radius R_1 is being pulled through a slightly larger tube of radius R_2. The gap between the two tubes is filled with a liquid of density ρ and viscosity μ. The fluid in the tube is prevented from leaving the tube by two seals at each end of the tube. These seals are made of Teflon, and thus there is negligible friction between the rod and the seal as the rod enters and leaves the tube. The length of the tube L is much larger that the gap (δ) between the tube and the rod: $R_2 - R_1 = \delta$. The outer tube is held in place by an external force.

(a) Draw a picture of, and calculate, the axial velocity profile, $V_x(y)$, in the gap between the rod and the tube ($y = 0$ at $r = R_1$ and $y = \delta$ at $r = R_2$). You may neglect the region very near the two seals where the flow is two-dimensional.
(b) Find the force (F) necessary for the rod to be pulled at a speed of U_0.

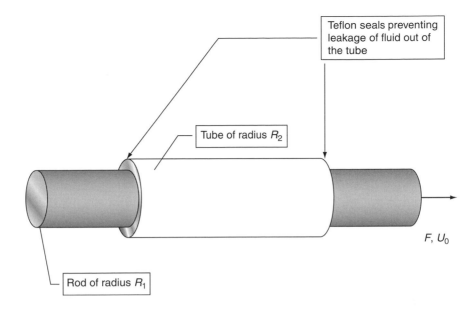

Teflon seals preventing leakage of fluid out of the tube

Tube of radius R_2

Rod of radius R_1

F, U_0

4.29. At most bifurcations of the airways in the lungs, the total cross-sectional area of the two daughter branches is larger than that of the parent branch. We are interested in determining how the rate of increase in cross-sectional area affects the average pressure gradient in the flow. To investigate this question, we build an experimental model as shown in the figure overleaf.

Here we have a circular duct of length L, for which $A(x) = A_0 \exp(x/\gamma)$, where $x = 0$ is the inlet to this duct. In our experiments, we will model just inspiration. Hence we will use a steady flow (Q) of air through the model. You may assume that the flow is not turbulent.

(a) Assuming that the flow can be modeled as inviscid and incompressible, predict the pressure change $P(x = 0) - P(x = L)$.

(b) Now, assuming that the flow can be modeled as dominated by viscous forces, predict the pressure change $P(x = 0) - P(x = L)$.

(c) Let $A_0 = 1$ cm^2, $L = 5$ cm and $Q = 2$ ml/s. The density of air is 0.0011 g/ml and the viscosity is 1.9×10^{-4} g/cm per s. For what range of numerical values of γ do you expect your answer to part (a) to give good predictions, and for what range of numerical values of γ do you expect your answer to part (b) to give good predictions?

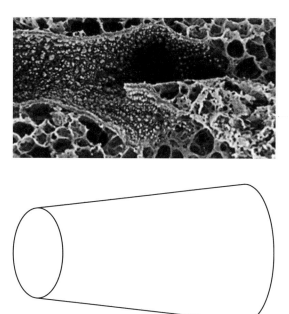

4.30. In the eye, a fluid called aqueous humor (of viscosity μ and density ρ) passes through a porous endothelium into a vessel known as Schlemm's canal. The flow rate of aqueous humor passing through this endothelium and entering the canal at location x, <u>per unit area of endothelium</u>, is denoted by $q(x)$ and is given by

$$q(x) = [P_0 - P(x)]/R_e$$

where $P(x)$ is the pressure in the canal at a location x, and P_0 and R_e are constants. The pressure at the exit of the canal ($x = \pm L$) is the episcleral venous pressure, which we will consider to be zero for this analysis.

While the canal is elliptical in cross-section (height a and depth into the page b), its major axis, b, is so much longer than its minor axis, a, that flow in Schlemm's canal can be approximated as flow between two parallel flat plates separated by a distance a. Owing to the small size of the canal and the low fluid velocity, the flow can be considered to be viscous, and inertial terms can be neglected. Consider the half of the canal segment shown in the figure with $0 < x < L$. The effect of gravity can be neglected.

(a)   Find an expression for dQ/dx where $Q(x)$ is the flow rate passing along the canal at a location x.

(b)   Find a differential equation that describes $P(x)$ in the canal in terms of μ, a, b, L, P_0, R_e, and ρ (not all of these parameters need necessarily be used).

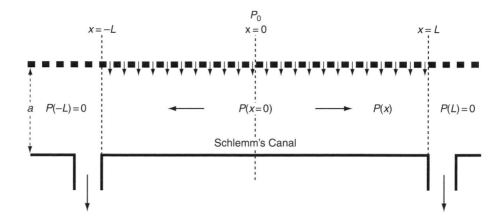

(c) Now assume that R_e is sufficiently large that the pressure inside the canal, $P(x)$, is much smaller than P_0. In this case, $q(x) = P_0/R_e$, a constant that is independent of x. Find the pressure $P(x = 0)$ in terms of μ, a, b, L, P_0, R_e, and ρ (not all of these parameters need necessarily be used).

(d) Give a criterion (again in terms of μ, a, b, L, P_0, R_e, and ρ – not all of these parameters need necessarily be used) that would allow you to decide whether the inertial forces are indeed negligible for this problem.

(e) Consider again part (c) but, in this case, without the assumption that $P(x) \ll P_0$. Find the total flow rate passing through this section of the canal for a given value of P_0.

4.31. In a new, minimally invasive procedure for coronary bypass, a needle or hollow "stent" of internal diameter 1.5 mm and length 1.5 cm is pushed through the wall of the left ventricle, forming a communicating channel from the ventricle to a point just distal to an obstruction in the coronary artery (see the figure). One end is open to the left ventricle while the other opens into the coronary artery. The complete arterial obstruction is on the left in the figure; the capillary bed is on the right. In preliminary experiments on this device, the flow rate through the stent varies as shown.

Use the following properties of blood: density 1.06 g/ml and viscosity 0.04 g/cm per s.

(a) Estimate the viscous pressure drop through the shunt (from point "1" to point "2") at a time during the acceleration phase of systole when the volume flow rate is 1 ml/s from the ventricle into the coronary artery. You may assume the flow to be quasi-steady and viscous-dominated.

(b) Describe how you would determine whether it is appropriate to neglect inertial effects in your estimate of the pressure drop and assume the flow to be viscous-dominated.

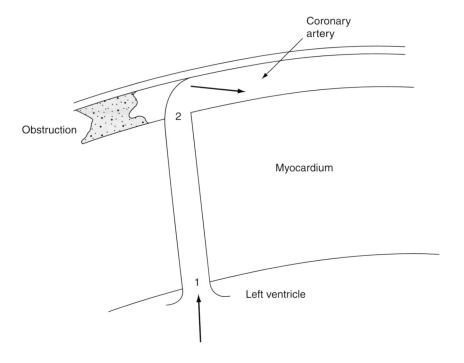

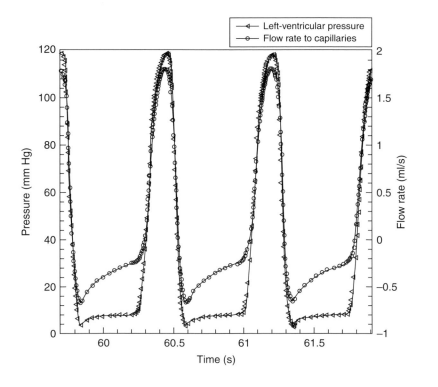

(c) Describe how you would determine whether it is appropriate to neglect the effects of temporal acceleration (unsteadiness) in your estimate of the pressure drop.

(d) If the conditions were such that unsteady inertia was significant inside the device, would the actual pressure difference across the stent be higher or lower than predicted in (a) during flow acceleration? Estimate by how much.

(e) Explain the time variation of the flow-rate trace in the context of the ventricular-pressure trace. Discuss both the magnitude and the direction of flow during systolc and diastolc.

(f) What information, in addition to what has been given above and in the figure, would one need in order to predict the time-varying flow-rate trace?

4.32. Many organs in the body accomplish transport through rhythmic, wave-like contractions of their walls, producing what is referred to as "peristaltic pumping." Consider here the pumping of a Newtonian fluid of viscosity μ through a tube of circular cross-section whose radius varies sinusoidally according to

$$a(z, t) = a_0 + b \sin \left[\frac{2\pi}{\lambda} (z - ct) \right]$$

where λ is the wavelength of the peristaltic wave, c is the wavespeed (as seen in a stationary reference frame), z is the axial position, and t is time. Note that we take $a_0 \ll \lambda$ so that appropriate simplifications can be made in the flow equations. You may assume the flow to be inertia-free. Note in this problem that the pressure-gradient term is the sum of an externally imposed gradient plus local pressure variations due to wall motion; we assume that the former contribution is constant in time, but clearly the latter contribution will be time-varying.

(a) You'll find it convenient to analyze this problem in a reference frame moving at the speed of the wave, c, so that the walls are stationary and the flow is steady. In that reference frame, obtain an expression for the velocity distribution, taking care to provide the correct boundary condition at the wall, in terms of the specified quantities as well as the unknown axial pressure gradient, dP/dz.

(b) Find expressions for the flow rate through the tube in the moving reference frame, Q', and the stationary frame, Q. Note that Q is time- and space-dependent, but Q' is not (this is important for the next two parts).

(c) Obtain an expression for the time-averaged flow rate $\overline{Q}$ produced by the peristaltic action.

(d) Integrate over one wavelength of the peristaltic wave to obtain an expression for the adverse (positive) pressure drop per wavelength $\Delta P_\lambda = \int_0^\lambda \frac{\partial P}{\partial z} dz$ to show that:

$$\Delta P_\lambda = \frac{4\mu c\lambda}{a_0^2 \, (1-\gamma^2)^{7/2}} \left[8\gamma^2 \left(1 - \frac{\gamma^2}{16}\right) - \frac{\overline{Q}}{\pi a_0^2 c}(2+3\gamma^2) \right]$$

Use this to obtain a final expression for $\overline{Q}$ with ΔP_λ as the only unknown. Note that the peristaltic wave is capable of generating flow against an adverse pressure gradient. What is the maximum value of ΔP_λ for which the flow is positive (in the direction of wave motion)?

Hint: the following integrals [19] will prove helpful:

$$\int_0^{2\pi} \frac{dy}{(1+\gamma \sin y)^2} = \frac{2\,\pi}{(1-\gamma^2)^{3/2}}$$

$$\int_0^{2\pi} \frac{dy}{(1+\gamma \sin y)^4} = \frac{\pi\,(2+3\gamma^2)}{(1-\gamma^2)^{7/2}}$$

4.33. Consider the inertia-free motion of fluid around a stationary spherical gas bubble or droplet of liquid that is immiscible in the flowing fluid. Let the fluid velocity far away from the bubble or droplet be in the axial direction and of magnitude V_∞.

(a) Seek a solution of Stokes' stream function $\psi = f(r)\sin^2\theta$ for flow past a sphere in the product form (from separation of variables), and show that $f(r) = Ar^4 + Br + Cr^2 + D/r$, where A, B, C, and D are constants of integration, is a solution.

(b) From the boundary conditions, determine the eight constants A_i, B_i, C_i, D_i, A_o, B_o, C_o, and D_o (i denotes inside fluid, o denotes outside fluid) in terms of V_∞, a (the sphere radius), μ_i and μ_o. (Hint: one of the eight boundary conditions involves the radial velocity of the fluid at $r = a$: what must be true of this velocity in order for the bubble surface to remain at $r = a$? Note also that the pressure inside the bubble at any location need not equal the pressure outside the bubble at that location.)

(c) Show that the drag force is given by

$$F_{\mathrm{D}} = 6\pi\mu a V_\infty \frac{1 + 2\mu_{\mathrm{o}}/(3\mu_{\mathrm{i}})}{1 + \mu_{\mathrm{o}}/\mu_{\mathrm{i}}}$$

(d) What are the limiting formulas for F_{D} if

    (i) $\mu_{\mathrm{i}} \gg \mu_{\mathrm{o}}$ (i.e. we have a solid sphere, or a liquid droplet in a gas) and

    (ii) $\mu_{\mathrm{i}} \ll \mu_{\mathrm{o}}$ (i.e. we have a gas bubble in a liquid).

Here are some relations that may help. For viscous flow around a sphere, the Stokes stream function in spherical coordinates ($\theta = 0$ is in the direction of flow) satisfies the following equation:

$$Q^2\psi = 0$$

where Q is a differential operator defined as

$$Q = \frac{\partial^2}{\partial r^2} + \frac{\sin\theta}{r^2}\frac{\partial}{\partial\theta}\left[\frac{1}{\sin\theta}\frac{\partial}{\partial\theta}\right]$$

and the Stokes equations reduce to

$$\frac{\partial P}{\partial r} = \frac{\mu}{r^2\sin\theta}\frac{\partial(Q\psi)}{\partial\theta}, \quad \frac{\partial P}{\partial\theta} = -\frac{\mu}{r\sin\theta}\frac{\partial(Q\psi)}{\partial r}$$

$$v_{\mathrm{r}} = -\frac{1}{r^2\sin\theta}\frac{\partial\psi}{\partial\theta}, \quad v_\theta = \frac{1}{r\sin\theta}\frac{\partial\psi}{\partial r}$$

5 Momentum boundary layers

(7 problems)

5.1. In an apparatus built in order to understand the influence of unsteady shear stress on endothelial cells, cells are plated onto the bottom surface of a rectangular channel that has a height of $h = 3$ mm and a width of $w = 10$ mm. The length of the channel is $L = 2$ cm.

  Saline (viscosity 0.01 g/cm per s and density 1 g/cm^3) flows in the channel with a flow rate of $Q = Q_0 \sin(\omega t)$; Q_0 is 2 ml/s. Roughly estimate the maximum shear stress acting on the cells for a low frequency of oscillation, $\omega = 0.01$ s^{-1}, and for a high frequency, $\omega = 10$ s^{-1}.

  You may neglect all entrance-length effects and thus assume that $\partial v_x/\partial x = 0$.

5.2. A fluid (density ρ and viscosity μ) enters a rectangular duct of width W and height h ($h \ll W$) at a flow rate Q. At the entrance, the velocity profile is uniform (constant) across the cross-section, but, as the fluid flows through the duct, the velocity profile changes to become Poiseuille (parabolic with a maximum velocity at the centerline). Determine the pressure drop (ΔP) between the entrance of the duct ($x = 0$) and the location at which the velocity profile first becomes Poiseuille ($x = L$) as a function of Q, h, W, ρ, and μ. (The flow is laminar and steady. W is the width of the duct into the page.)

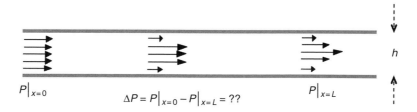

$P|_{x=0}$

$\Delta P = P|_{x=0} - P|_{x=L} = ??$

$P|_{x=L}$

h

5.3. A cone-and-plate viscometer is a device that is used to measure the viscosity of different fluids. It has found many biological applications. In such a device, a cone (of very gradual angle α) is rotated above a flat plate with a very small gap between the two surfaces. Owing to the angle, this gap increases linearly with radius (see the figure). The advantage of such a device is that the shear rate is everywhere the same. This is important because many physiological fluids show a decreased viscosity with increasing shear rate. Let the angle $\alpha \ll 1$. You may ignore the flow in the edge gap.

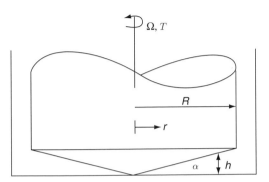

(a) Show that the shear is everywhere essentially independent of location under steady-state conditions.

(b) When the device is first started, there is a period of time before the shear stress everywhere reaches its steady-state value. Estimate this time-scale (an exact calculation is not necessary) if a fluid that has a viscosity similar to that of water is tested.

(c) Assume that the fluid being tested in the viscometer is everywhere homogeneous but non-Newtonian (the viscosity depends on the shear rate). From experimental measurements of the applied torque (T) and the rotational speed of the cone (Ω), show how to determine the effective viscosity at the applied shear rate.

5.4. Blood flow in blood vessels is pulsatile. Under some conditions, the velocity profile of the blood will be a Poiseuille profile modulated in time, whereas under other conditions inertial effects can become important.

(a) Consider pulsatile flow of blood with viscosity μ and density ρ with a flow rate of blood $Q(t) = Q_0 \sin(\omega t)$ in a vessel of radius R. The blood vessel can be assumed to be sufficiently long that entrance effects can be ignored for all parts of this problem. Find the conditions under which the flow can be assumed to be inertia-free and thus to have a time-modulated Poiseuille velocity profile.

(b) If this inertia-free flow is being driven by a pressure gradient $dP/dx = G_0 \sin(\omega t + \delta)$, determine δ, the phase shift between the flow and the pressure gradient.

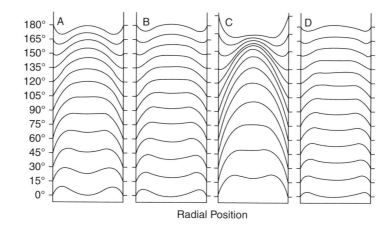

Radial Position

(c) Assume that the conditions that you determined in part (a) of this question are not met, so that inertia in the flow is now important. Are there conditions under which the effects of viscosity can be ignored? If so, what are they?

(d) Consider a flow in which viscous and inertial effects are both important. Near the wall, a boundary layer will develop. Estimate the thickness of this boundary layer.

(e) Now consider the core of the flow outside this boundary layer. If this flow is being driven by a pressure gradient $dP/dx = G_0 \sin(\omega t + \delta)$, determine δ.

(f) Consider the figure showing the velocity profile inside the vessel for oscillatory flow at different times in the cycle (phase from 0° to 180°). Rank these profiles in terms of the parameter that you determined for part (a). Each panel represents a different flow condition. Profiles within each panel are taken at 12 equally spaced times during half of an oscillatory flow cycle. From [3].

5.5. The blood flow entering an artery is pulsatile such that $Q(t) = Q_0 + Q_1 \sin(\omega t)$. While the arteries can change their dimensions with pressure, they are much stiffer than veins and thus, to a first approximation, can be considered to have a constant diameter. Consider a vessel with a diameter D. Let the magnitudes of Q_0 and Q_1 be comparable.

(a)   How does Q vary with x at each instant in time?

(b)   The characteristics of the pulsatile flow change dramatically as the blood passes from large vessels to small vessels. In the large vessels, the flow behaves as if it were inviscid. What dimensionless parameter(s) determine in which vessels such an assumption would be correct?

(c)   For the large vessels in which the flow behaves as if it were inviscid, (i) calculate dP/dx and (ii) draw the velocity profile.

(d)   In the very small vessels, viscous forces dominate. What are the conditions that would be required for the dimensionless parameter(s) you determined for part (b)?

(e)   For these viscous conditions, (i) calculate dP/dx and (ii) draw the velocity profile.

(f)   Now consider a vessel such that both inertial and viscous forces are important. Sketch the velocity profiles at four times during the cycle: at $0°$ (just starting), $90°$, $180°$, and $270°$. Let $Q_0 = Q_1$.

5.6. The semicircular canals in your ears work by sensing motion of endo-lymph inside the canals, using a tissue called the ampulla, and translating this into information about acceleration of the head. Shown in the first

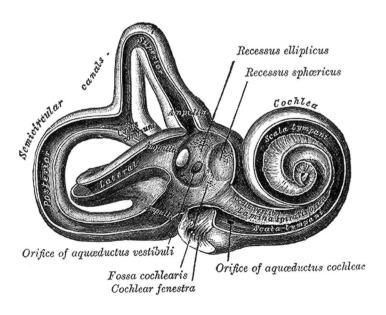

Recessus ellipticus
Recessus sphœricus

Orifice of aquœductus vestibuli
Fossa cochlearis
Cochlear fenestra
Orifice of aquœductus cochleœ

figure below (from [4]) are these three semicircular canals (posterior, superior, and lateral), each with an ampulla. When the head moves in any direction, flow is generated in one of these canals, with an ampulla deforming to allow flow.

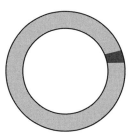

To model flow in the posterior canal, consider it to be a circular thin tube of length $L = 20$ mm and tube diameter $2R = 0.3$ mm (see the second figure, above) with a deformable membrane (the ampulla) at one location (shown in dark gray). Note that we have ignored the connection between the posterior canal and the superior canal known as the "crus commune." Let the flow rate (Q) in the canal (relative to the moving canal walls) generated by head motion be $Q = Q_0 \sin(\omega t)$. We want to find the pressure difference (ΔP) acting across the membrane as a function of time. Let the fluid in the canal have the same density (ρ) and viscosity (μ) as water at 37 °C.

(a) Find $\Delta P(t)$ in terms of given parameters (Q_0, ω, μ, ρ, R, and L) when the frequency of head motion is very low (ω approaching 0).
(b) Find $\Delta P(t)$ in terms of the given parameters (Q_0, ω, μ, ρ, R, and L) when the frequency of head motion is very high (ω approaching infinity).
(c) For what frequencies do you expect you answer to part (b) to be correct?
(d) The upper limit of frequency to which the endolymph can respond to head motion is roughly $\omega = 40$ Hz (251 radians/s) with a corresponding flow of $Q_0 = 0.06$ ml/s. Roughly estimate the magnitude of the shear stresses on the walls of the canal at this frequency.

5.7. A thin-walled pipe 2 cm in diameter and 120 cm long is towed through still oil ($\rho = 0.85$ g/cm^3, $\mu = 11$ g/cm per s) at 80 cm/s. The direction of towing is parallel to the long axis of the pipe.

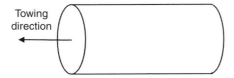

Make as accurate an estimation as you can of the total force necessary to tow this pipe. Clearly state any assumptions that you make. You may assume that the flow outside of the pipe behaves like flow over a flat plate.

6 Piping systems, friction factors, and drag coefficients

(6 problems)

6.1. Consider the case of mitral regurgitation. If the connection between the ventricle and atrium can be treated as a hole of diameter 0.2 cm, estimate the rate of leakage from the ventricle into the atrium at a time when the ventricular pressure is 100 mm Hg and the atrial pressure is 10 mm Hg. (Note that 760 mm Hg = 1.01×10^5 Pa.) You can neglect unsteadiness. Use a blood density of 1.06 g/cm^3 and a viscosity of 0.04 g/cm per s.

6.2. One way to measure cardiac output is to inject a tracer into the blood stream and watch how quickly it disperses. This requires a rapid injection of tracer, which is often done by using a tracer-injector device.

One such injector consists of a large syringe that creates a pressure of 300 kPa. The tracer flows from the injector through 4 m of smooth plastic tubing of internal diameter 3 mm, then through a smooth 23-gauge needle (4 cm long, internal diameter 0.455 mm) before entering a peripheral vein where the pressure is 10 mm Hg (1.333 kPa). Neglecting minor losses and the height difference between the injector and the vein, what will the flow rate of tracer be?

Note that <u>iteration</u> is required in order to solve this question. The physical properties for the tracer are $\rho = 1000$ kg/m^3 and $v = \mu/\rho = 1.0 \times 10^{-6}$ m^2/s.

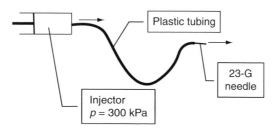

6.3. A cyclist rides her bike for a distance d due north, then turns around and rides due south to return to her starting point. Neglect rolling resistance and assume that the cycling route is on flat, level ground.

(a) If she rides at constant speed V for the entire trip, compute her total energy expenditure and average power output as a function of her drag coefficient, C_D, frontal area, A, and other relevant parameters. Recall that power is work done per unit time.

(b) The next day she does the same ride at the same constant speed V, even though a steady wind blows due north at speed U for the entire trip. Is her average power output on the windy day the same, less than, or greater than her average power output on the still day? What is the difference, if any, between her power outputs on the two days?

6.4. A stent is a device that is inserted into a diseased artery to hold the artery open. The stent consists of cylindrical metal wires that form a network that is expanded against the artery wall from the inside. Suppose a stent is placed in a coronary artery such that it occludes a side-branch artery that has diameter $D_{SB} = 1$ mm.

(a) Estimate the pressure drop due to the stent wires as blood enters the side branch at $Q_{SB} = 0.3$ ml/s. The diameter of the stent wires is $D_W = 0.15$ mm, and the total length of wires crossing the branch mouth is 2.4 mm. State relevant assumptions. The graph of C_D vs. Re_D for flow over a cylinder may be helpful (Re is based on cylinder diameter; data from Rosendahl [5]). C_D is based on the projected area of the cylinder.

Stent Entering Artery

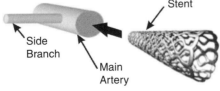

Image courtesy of Sono-Tek Corporation

Stent as seen from Side branch

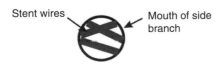

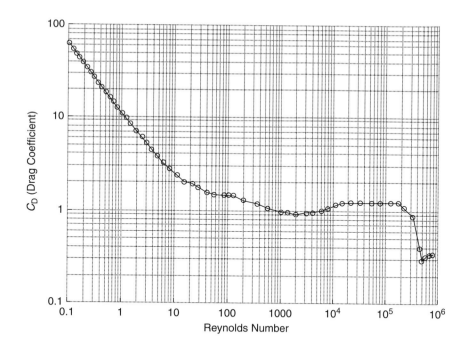

(b) Compare this with the time-averaged pressure drop over the length of the 22-mm-long side-branch artery.

The properties of the blood are $\mu = 3.5$ cP and $\rho = 1.05$ g/cm^3.

6.5. As part of a refrigeration system to be used for a new X-ray CT imaging system, water is pumped around a loop containing two heat exchangers. Each heat exchanger has a minor loss coefficient of $K = 17.4$, based on the water velocity in the 10-cm-diameter inlet to the heat exchanger. All other minor losses sum to a total loss coefficient of 2.5. The total length of piping is 34 m, with a diameter of 10 cm and an absolute roughness of 0.01 mm. You may neglect height variations through the system and changes in physical properties due to temperature variations.

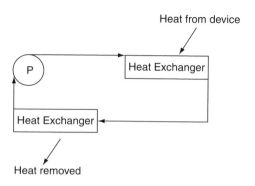

If the pump has a head-discharge curve of the form $H = 100 - Q^2$, with H in meters and Q in m^3/s, what is the resulting flow rate? The solution requires iteration (write the solution as $Q = f(Q)$, then guess a value of Q and solve for a new guess for Q; continue until the solution converges).

The physical properties of water are $\rho = 1000$ kg/m^3 and $v = \mu/\rho = 1.0 \times 10^{-6}$ m^2/s.

6.6. It is of interest to design a system to automate the process of injecting fluid into a vein using a needle. At $t = 0$, assume the the syringe plunger is to be pushed such that flow out of the needle is Q_0 (constant) for $t > 0$. The relative motion between the plunger and the syringe barrel can be assumed to be frictionless. We want to know how much force we need to apply to the plunger in order to move it relative to the stationary syringe barrel.

The fluid has a viscosity of $\mu = 0.01$ g/cm per s and a density of $\rho = 1$ g/cm^3. You may assume that the internal diameter of the needle (d_n) is much less than that of the syringe barrel ($d_n \ll d_p$), and that the venous pressure is equal to atmospheric pressure. All answers should be given in symbolic form unless noted otherwise. However, if you need to evaluate the magnitude of any terms, you may use the following parameter values: $d_n = 0.5$ mm, $d_p = 20$ mm, $Q_0 = 0.1$ cm^3/s, $L_1 = 2$ cm, and $L_2 = 5$ cm.

(a) First assume inviscid flow and steady-state conditions. Find the pressure in the syringe barrel (at the plunger).
(b) Now assume viscous-dominated flow and steady-state conditions. Find the pressure in the syringe barrel (at the plunger).
(c) For this part, consider the parameter values given above. Find the steady-state pressure in the syringe barrel (at the plunger). Give a numerical answer.
(d) For the conditions of part (c), determine how much force needs to be applied to push the plunger and keep the flow rate constant at Q_0.

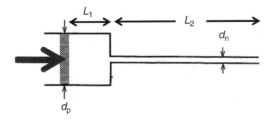

7 Problems involving surface tension
(6 problems)

7.1. Consider a small spherical bubble of radius R of air in a large liquid volume.

(a) Show that the energy required to expand this sphere by a *small* amount ΔR is $2\sigma\,\Delta V/R$. Here ΔV is the increase in volume and σ is the interfacial tension.

(b) Estimate the cycle-averaged power required in order to overcome alveolar surface tension during normal breathing. Take $R = 150$ μm, $\sigma = 25$ dyne/cm, and a breathing rate of 12 breaths per minute, and let the tidal volume be 500 ml.

(c) The figure shows an idealized pressure–volume curve for a cat's lung during normal breathing. Repeat the calculation above for the cat lung, where $R = 80$ μm and $\sigma = 35$ dyne/cm, with a breathing rate of 20 breaths per minute, and let the tidal volume be 25 ml. Compare this calculated value with a *rough* estimate of the power obtained from the figure. (Take the beginning of normal inspiration to occur at 105 ml.) Is surface tension or lung-tissue elasticity the dominant restoring force in the cat lung? (Modified from Ethier and Simmons [2].)

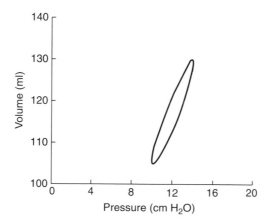

7.2. As a neutrophil (initially spherical of radius R_N) passes through the capillary bed of the lung, it encounters a narrow capillary segment with a radius smaller than its own radius, $R_C = R_N/2$. Consequently, it needs to deform in order to pass through.

You may model the neutrophil as a membrane with constant tension σ (but negligible bending stiffness) filled with a Newtonian fluid of viscosity μ_N. Any effects of an internal cytoskeleton (other than the membrane-associated cortex) can be neglected. Obtain an expression for the minimum, critical pressure drop across the capillary segment necessary to cause the neutrophil to enter and pass through, given sufficient time to do so.

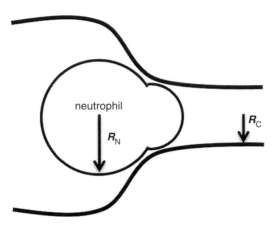

7.3. Consider water (at 20 °C) coming steadily out of a small faucet vertically into the air as a thin jet. Let the jet narrow from a diameter of 2 mm to a diameter of 1 mm over a distance of 4 cm. Ignoring viscous effects (and any instabilities), calculate the flow rate coming out of the faucet.

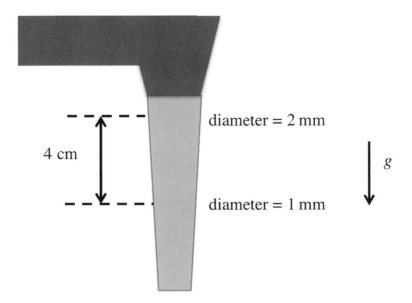

7.4. The pulmonary airways are lined with liquid that is thought to constitute a thin, continuous layer extending from the lung periphery to the trachea. This layer ranges in thickness from less than 1 μm in the smallest airways to about 10 μm in the trachea. The air–liquid interface of this layer has a surface tension that is influenced by the presence of a surfactant, which is produced in the alveolar region (the ends of the airways) and is likely to be present, but in reduced concentrations, further up the airway tree. In this problem, you will consider the flows induced in this thin liquid layer due to the presence of a gradient in surface tension that exists due to this difference in surfactant concentration as well as other factors.

Assume the layer of liquid behaves as a Newtonian fluid with a density of 1 g/cm^3 and a viscosity of 1 cP, has a uniform thickness of 5 μm, and is acted upon by a uniform surface-tension gradient of 0.2 N/m^2 in the lower airways (with the surface tension decreasing from larger airways to smaller airways). The radii of these airways are much larger than the thickness of the layer, and can be assumed to be constant over short segments of airways.

(a) Neglecting gravity and the effects of air motion, determine the maximum speed at which the liquid is propelled due to the gradient in surface tension. The surface-tension gradient exerts a shear stress on the surface of the liquid equal in magnitude to the gradient, $d\sigma/dx$, where σ is the surface tension. Compare this with the speed at which cilia propel the liquid, about 2×10^{-4} m/s.

(b) Now include the effect of gravity (assuming the airway is vertical), and determine how this affects this surface velocity.

(c) Find a dimensionless variable that characterizes when gravity is important in this calculation.

7.5. Consider a membrane of thickness $l = 10$ μm, with a number of small holes of varying size (radius) passing through this membrane. Assume that the size distribution of these pores is unknown. As a method to determine the pore-size distribution (before the advent of electron microscopy), Huggert [6] developed a clever scheme whereby he perfused the membrane first with water and then with isobutyl alcohol. This alcohol exhibits a surface tension toward water of $\sigma = 23$ dyne/cm and has a viscosity of 0.02 g/cm per s. He measured the flow of alcohol through the membrane at low pressure and then at a set of gradually increasing pressures. Note that pores whose opening pressure exceeds the driving pressure will not carry any flow; as the driving pressure increases, more pores will be recruited for flow. The opening pressure for a pore can be computed from Laplace's law.

The curve shown in the figure was the result. Assuming that the pore size and membrane thickness do not vary with pressure, find the pore-size distribution. In

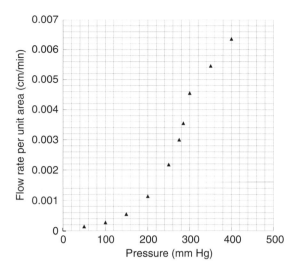

solving this problem, you will find it convenient to work with a function $n(r)$ that describes the number of pores per unit membrane area, such that $n(r)dr$ is the number of pores/area in the interval r to $r + dr$.

7.6. The airways of the lung are coated with a very thin liquid lining. In the upper airways this fluid is continuously moved upward toward the mouth by the cilia. In the lowest airways there are few ciliated cells, and the fluid motion is determined by a balance between surface-tension forces and, to a much lesser extent, by gravity.

Since the airways become progressively smaller on going from one generation to the next, surface-tension forces would be expected to pull this liquid into the lung, eventually filling the alveoli. Assume that, in the small airways, the average airway radius is $R = 0.05$ mm, the surface tension is 25 dyne/cm, and the liquid lining thickness is $h = 5$ µm, and that the airways decrease in radius with increasing airway length by 0.015 mm/mm (you may assume that $h \ll R$). Assume further that the liquid behaves as a Newtonian fluid with a density of 1 g/cm^3 and a viscosity of 1 cP.

Assuming that this airway is vertical, calculate what the gradient in surface tension must be such that there is no net drainage of fluid down toward the alveoli. Note that the surface-tension gradient affects both the gradient of pressure in the liquid layer and also the shear stress at the air–liquid interface. You may neglect gravity and the effect of air motion in the airway.

8 Non-Newtonian blood flow

(10 problems)

8.1. Blood is really a non-Newtonian fluid that has both solid-like and fluid-like characteristics. At high shear stress, blood behaves somewhat like a Newtonian fluid (with a viscosity about five times that of plasma, or 0.035 g/cm per s), whereas at low shear stresses blood acts like a solid. The shear stress at which blood starts to flow is quite low, approximately 0.05 dyne/cm^2. (This is really a simplification: blood really behaves as a Casson fluid with non-Newtonian character even for shear rates above the yield stress.)

(a) For an arteriole of diameter 200 μm and length 500 μm, determine how large the pressure drop would have to be before blood would just begin to flow through this blood vessel.

(b) Now let the pressure drop driving flow through this arteriole be twice as high as that calculated in part (a), and find the rate of blood flow through this arteriole.

8.2. A Casson fluid (like blood), described by the constitutive relations

$$\tau^{1/2} = \begin{cases} 0, & \text{for } \tau < \tau_y \\ \tau_y^{1/2} + K\dot{\gamma}^{1/2}, & \text{for } \tau > \tau_y \end{cases}$$

where τ_y is the yield stress, is placed between two parallel plates, and a constant shear stress τ is applied to the upper plate while the bottom plate is held stationary

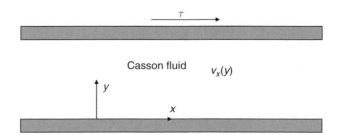

(with $dP/dx = 0$). Here $\dot{\gamma}$ is the shear rate, dv_x/dy. Sketch the velocity profile $v_x(y)$ for (i) when $\tau < \tau_y$ and (ii) when $\tau > \tau_y$, and find the effective viscosity for case (ii).

8.3. Consider steady laminar blood flow in a vessel of radius R. Model this flow as that of a Casson fluid with a yield stress of τ_y (see the constitutive relation in the previous problem). A differential force balance and solution of the resulting differential equation with this constitutive relation (and the no-slip boundary condition) yield the following axial velocity distribution:

$$v_z(r) = -\frac{R^2}{4K^2}\frac{dp}{dz}\left\{1 - \left(\frac{r}{R}\right)^2 - \frac{8}{3}\sqrt{\frac{R_c}{R}}\left[1 - \left(\frac{r}{R}\right)^{3/2}\right] + \frac{2R_c}{R}\left(1 - \frac{r}{R}\right)\right\}(r > R_c)$$

where R_c is the radius of the non-flowing "core," i.e. the region where the local shear stress is less than the yield stress.

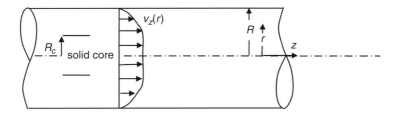

(a)   Show that R_c can be found as

$$R_c = \frac{2\tau_y}{-dp/dz}$$

(b)   Show that the flow rate Q in this vessel is

$$Q = \frac{\pi R^4}{8K^2}\left(-\frac{dp}{dz}\right)\left[1 - \frac{16}{7}\left(\frac{R_c}{R}\right)^{1/2} + \frac{4}{3}\left(\frac{R_c}{R}\right) - \frac{1}{21}\left(\frac{R_c}{R}\right)^4\right]$$

(c)   Explain the limits when $R_c = 0$ and when $R_c = R$. What physical interpretation do you give to the parameter K?

(Note that, for Problems 8.4–8.8, the flow rate for a Casson fluid in a tube is that given in this problem.)

8.4. Blood with a Casson yield stress $\tau_y = 0.2$ dyne/cm^2 is forced through a series of tubes of different radii (see the table overleaf). The same pressure gradient of

2.0 dyne/cm^3 is used for all tubes, and the flow rates shown in the table are taken from experimental measurements. Compute the blood's Casson coefficient K from these data. Because of noise in the experimental measurements, for a reliable estimate for K one needs to consider information from all four tubes.

Tube radius (cm)	Blood flow rate (cm^3/s)
1.0	6.0
2.0	171
3.0	1000
4.0	3700

8.5. Blood flows steadily in a tube of radius 1 cm due to a pressure gradient of 0.4 dyne/cm^3. Treating the blood as a Casson fluid with yield stress 0.06 dyne/cm^2, what percentage of the total volume flow rate is due to blood traveling in the central non-flowing "core" of the flow? From [2].

8.6. Blood from two different patients is to be tested by having it flow through a long straight tube of length 10 cm and internal diameter 6 mm. A pressure drop of 50 dyne/cm^2 is imposed from one end of the tube to the other, and the resulting blood flow rate Q is measured.

(a) If the blood from patient A has a yield shear stress of 0.08 dyne/cm^2 and the blood from patient B has a yield shear stress of 0.12 dyne/cm^2, predict the ratio Q_A/Q_B. Assume that the blood from these two patients follows identical Casson rheology, with the exception of the difference in yield stress.

(b) Now compare these flow rates with those expected for the case of a fluid with a yield shear stress of zero (a Newtonian fluid) with a viscosity of K^2. All other parameters of the flow (pressure gradient, etc.) are identical to those in part (a). From [2].

8.7. Flowing blood is frequently modeled as a Casson fluid, with a yield stress for fluid motion and shear-thinning behavior with increasing shear rate. The following constitutive law relating the shear stress τ to the shear rate dv_z/dr describes such behavior:

$$K^2 = \begin{cases} \infty, & |\tau| < \tau_0 \\ \dfrac{(|\tau|^{1/2} - \tau_y^{1/2})^2}{|dv_z/dr|}, & |\tau| > \tau_0 \end{cases}$$

where τ_y is the yield stress for fluid motion, K is a measure of the "viscosity" of the fluid and $v_z(r)$ is the velocity of the blood in the axial direction at a radial location r. However, blood can also be modeled as a Bingham fluid that has a yield stress, but does not exhibit shear-thinning behavior. Its constitutive law is somewhat simpler:

$$K^2 = \begin{cases} \infty, & |\tau| < \tau_0 \\ \dfrac{(|\tau| - \tau_y)}{|dv_z/dr|}, & |\tau| > \tau_0 \end{cases}$$

For flow in a circular tube of radius R, compare the flow rate of a Bingham fluid with that of a Casson fluid if each has the same value of K and the same yield stress. Be careful about the signs of the shear stress and velocity gradient.

8.8. Biomedical engineers have developed perfluorocarbon-emulsion blood substitutes that have the oxygen-carrying capacity of blood but can be stored for long periods. The graph shows rheological measurements for whole blood, and for blood diluted with two such emulsions (modified from Jouan-Hureaux *et al.* [7]). The table below shows numerical values taken from the graph for low shear rates. The effective viscosity is the ratio of the measured shear stress to the applied shear rate. You may assume that each mixture behaves as a Casson fluid.

	Effective viscosity (cP)	
Shear rate (1/s)	Mixture A	Mixture B
0.2	32.10	18.83
0.5	23.29	14.02
0.95	18.84	11.66
3.3	12.58	8.58

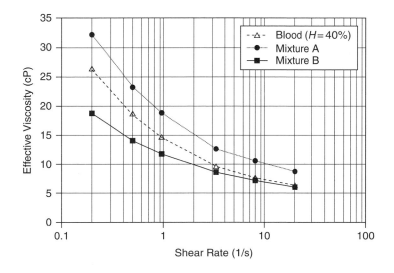

(a) Describe how you would use the data in the table to estimate the yield stress and viscosity coefficient for mixture A and for mixture B. Your explanation will ideally include a diagram, at least one formula, and a suitable amount of explanatory text.

(b) Show that the data given in the table for mixture B are consistent with a Casson yield stress of $\tau_{y,B} = 0.008$ dyne/cm^2 and a Casson coefficient of $K_B^2 = 6.0$ cP.

(c) If mixture A and mixture B are driven by a pressure gradient of 0.4 dyne/cm^3 through identical long cylindrical tubes of diameter 1 cm, which mixture will have the greater flow rate, and by how much?

8.9. It has been observed that, in small blood vessels (i.e. those smaller than a few hundred micrometers in diameter), the tube hematocrit H_T (the volume of red blood cells (RBCs) in a blood vessel divided by the blood volume in the blood vessel) is less than the hematocrit in the general circulation (H). This is called the Fåhræus effect, and is due to the plasma-skimming layer, a thin layer very near the wall where RBCs are excluded due to their size and to the tendency of lift forces to move RBCs away from the wall.

(a) Assuming a Poiseuille velocity profile, find a relationship between the thickness of the plasma-skimming layer, δ, and H_R, where $H_R = H_T/H$. You may assume that there are no RBCs in the plasma-skimming layer, and that they are uniformly distributed through the rest of the plasma in the tube.

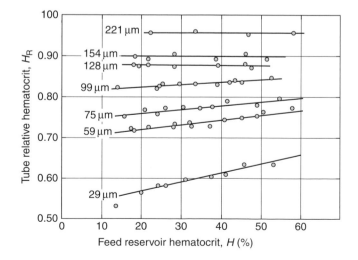

(b) The figure [8] on the previous page shows how H_R depends on the feed reservoir hematocrit (H) for vessels of different diameters. Calculate the effect of vessel diameter on δ at reservoir feed hematocrits of 20% and 50%.

(c) Speculate as to why increasing the feed reservoir hematocrit has an effect on δ.

8.10. In small blood vessels we know that the hematocrit is small near the wall and larger near the center of the vessel. Blood viscosity is affected by hematocrit, and hence we expect the local blood viscosity to vary with radial position in such a vessel. In 1956, Kynch [9] extended Einstein's 1906 result to show that the relationship between viscosity, μ, and particle solid fraction, H, could be expressed by

$$\mu = \mu_0\left(1 + \frac{5}{2}H + \frac{25}{4}H^2\right)$$

where μ_0 is the viscosity of the suspending fluid (plasma in our case). (Note that this is valid only up to solid fractions of about 30%. Note also that, in blood, the solid fraction is equivalent to the hematocrit.)

(a) Suppose that experimental measurements show that the velocity profile in a vessel of radius R can be empirically fit by the equation

$$u(r) = -\frac{dp}{dx}\frac{R^2}{6\mu_0}\left[1 - \left(\frac{r}{R}\right)^3\right]$$

where (x, r) are cylindrical coordinates for the vessel. From this empirical fit, and using the expression for viscosity given above, derive an expression for the hematocrit in the vessel as a function of the radial position, r. You may assume that the blood acts as a Newtonian fluid whose viscosity varies with position.

(b) Comment on the expression you derived in part (a). Does it seem realistic?

9 Dimensional analysis

(12 problems)

9.1. Fluid often passes through pores in cell membranes or cell layers. The dimensions are small and the velocities low, so viscous forces dominate (low Reynolds number). Use dimensional analysis, or an approximate method of analysis based on the viscous flow equations, to determine the scaling law that expresses the dependence of the pressure drop across a pore (ΔP) on the flow rate through it (Q). The other parameters that are given include the pore radius, R, and the viscosity of the fluid, μ. The membrane itself should be considered infinitesimally thin so that its thickness does not influence the pressure drop.

9.2. Using a stroboscope, it has been observed that freely falling water drops vibrate. The characteristic time for this vibration does not depend on the viscosity of the water (except for very, very small drops). Determine what parameters you expect this vibration time to depend on, and find a relationship between the vibration time and these parameters. Estimate the characteristic vibration time for a water droplet of diameter 2 mm at a temperature of 25° C. (Hint: this time-scale is the same for a droplet inside of a rocket in space as it is for a droplet falling on the Earth.)

9.3. The mouse is now being widely used as a model of cardiovascular disease in humans. Researchers have decided to study blood flow patterns in the mouse aorta. To do so, they build a five-times-larger scale model of the aorta (all linear dimensions increased five-fold), attach it to a pulsatile pump to simulate the heart, and use a model fluid with the properties shown in the table below. Because it is known that disease development depends in part on the shear stress, τ, exerted by flowing blood on the endothelial cells that line the arteries, they wish to measure this quantity.

Quantity	Mouse	Five-times-larger model
Heart rate, HR (beats/min)	650	?
Cardiac output, Q (l/min)	0.026	?
Fluid density, ρ (g/cm^3)	1.05	1.8
Fluid viscosity, μ (cP)	3.5	17

(a) Confirm that three Π-groups can be formed from the relevant parameters in this problem. Note that not all of the relevant parameters are listed in the table.

(b) Find these Π-groups.

(c) What "heart rate" and flow rate should be used in the five-times-larger model so as to match the situation in the mouse aorta?

(d) If a shear stress of 35 dyne/cm^2 is measured at a certain location in the five-times-larger model, what will the corresponding shear stress be at the corresponding location in the mouse aorta?

9.4. There is currently a great deal of interest in delivering drugs (e.g. insulin) by inhalation, thus avoiding the need for their injection (e.g. [10]). Aerosol droplets of density ρ_I and diameter D containing the drug would be inhaled and reach the small airways, where they would be absorbed into the blood. One problem is that droplets can have a hard time following tortuous pathways in the lungs, and run into airway walls before reaching their target destination. This depends on the speed of the air, v_{Air}, as well as on the viscosity and density of the air, μ_{Air} and ρ_{Air}. Droplets can also sediment out of the air stream, depending on the gravitational acceleration, g.

(a) Determine how many Π-groups can be formed from these parameters.

(b) Find these Π-groups.

(c) The efficiency of delivery, e, is a fourth Π-group, so that $e = \text{fn}(\Pi_1, \Pi_2, \Pi_3)$. A five-times-larger scale model of the large airways of the lung is built and is to be tested using small spheres instead of droplets. The spheres have diameter five times that of the droplets and density three times that of the droplets. What fluid density, viscosity, and speed (ρ_{Model}, μ_{Model}, and v_{Model}), should be used in this five-times-larger model? Express your answers in terms of ratios ρ_{Model}/ρ_{Air}, μ_{Model}/μ_{Air}, and v_{Model}/v_{Air}.

9.5. Fluid drainage from an edematous tissue is driven by the swelling pressure within the tissue, which forces the water out of the interstitium and into the capillaries. On the other hand, fluid drainage is opposed by the hydrodynamic resistance of the interstitium, such that the net rate at which the tissue drains results from a balance between tissue swelling and interstitial hydrodynamic resistance. We can characterize this interstitial resistance by a parameter that we call the tissue resistivity, which is defined as $T_R = \mu/K$, where μ is the viscosity of the draining fluid and K is the interstitial permeability

The time-scale for edema clearance, τ, is expected to depend on the tissue resistivity and the size of the region to be drained (which is characterized by the domain radius R) but should be independent of the magnitude of the initial swelling pressure in the tissue (i.e. τ is the time constant for decay of the swelling pressure). This time-scale will be affected also by the tissue elasticity γ. If a bruise has a characteristic size of $R = 5.5 \times 10^{-2}$ cm and the other quantities have the values $K = 8 \times 10^{-14}$ cm^2, $\gamma = 4540$ dyne/cm^2, and $\mu = 0.01$ g/cm per s, estimate the time-scale τ for persistence of this bruise (assuming that reduction of swelling is the time-limiting process).

9.6. The lung is an elastic structure that is periodically filled by air. This filling and emptying during normal tidal breathing is driven by variations in pressure in the pleural cavity surrounding the lung. These variations in pressure, ΔP, depend on the frequency of breathing, f, the air density, ρ (but not the air viscosity, μ), the volume of the lung, V, the tidal volume, ΔV, and the elastic modulus of the lung tissue, E (Young's modulus). In normal human breathing, the tidal volume is 400 ml, and the frequency of breathing is 14 breaths per minute. You may assume that the elastic modulus of the rat lung is similar to that of the human lung.

(a) Rats are frequently used in experiments to study pulmonary function. A human lung is roughly 500 times larger than a rat lung, by volume. If a rat lung is put in an experimental apparatus that controls pleural pressure variations, what tidal volume and what frequency of breathing should be used if the experiments are to model human tidal breathing?

(b) If the ΔP in these experiments on rat lungs was measured to be 4 cm H$_2$O, predict what value of ΔP would be expected in the pleural space of human lungs during normal tidal breathing.

9.7. The diffusion of substances such as platelets and macromolecules in the blood is enhanced by the complicated fluid motions surrounding the red blood cells (RBCs). This enhanced diffusion coefficient (D_{eff}) is a function of the effective radius of the RBCs ($a = 4$ μm) and the shear rate in the blood. Estimate whether this might have a significant effect on the transport of oxygen ($D = 2 \times 10^{-5}$ cm^2/s), a typical macromolecule (albumin, $D = 8 \times 10^{-7}$ cm^2/s), and platelets ($D = 1 \times 10^{-9}$ cm^2/s) in a blood vessel of radius $R = 0.05$ mm carrying blood at a flow rate of $Q = 1$ μl/min.

9.8. In some diseases, liquid can accumulate in the airways and trap bubbles. It is then more difficult for air to flow through these airways.

Consider a bubble of volume V trapped in an airway of radius R as shown in the figure. We are interested in determining how much the presence of this bubble increases the pressure drop for flow. The effects of gravity can be neglected. The viscosity and density of the air in the bubble are also negligible. You may assume that the flow of airway liquid is sufficiently slow and the viscosity of this liquid is sufficiently high that inertial effects can be neglected.

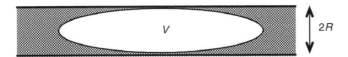

Let the airway liquid have density ρ, viscosity μ, and surface tension (with respect to air) σ. Experiments are done measuring the pressure drop (ΔP, the pressure behind the bubble minus the pressure in front of the bubble) on a bubble moving through tubes of different radii (R) at a bubble velocity of U. It is found that ΔP is proportional to $\sigma^{1/3}$ and is inversely proportional to R (for bubbles large enough to fill the tube).

Consider two airways, the larger one twice the radius of the smaller ($R_1 = 2R_2$), each with a bubble and each with the same airway liquid. The bubble in the larger airway has four times the volume of that in the smaller airway ($V_1 = 4V_2$). If the pressure drop across a bubble in each of the two airways is the same, what will the ratio of bubble velocities in the two airways be (U_1/U_2)?

9.9. In some forms of airway disease, the airways become flooded with liquid, and bubbles can become trapped in these airways. When the bubbles are then driven by buoyancy through the airways, shear stresses are generated on the airway wall, and it has been hypothesized that the epithelium covering the airways can be damaged by this shear stress.

The problem of analyzing the motion of a long bubble through a small airway (see the figure below) is complicated. One possible way to address the problem is to build an experimental model, measure the velocity at which the bubble moves

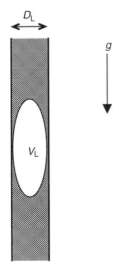

through the model system, and then use the result to determine the velocity at which a bubble might pass through a fluid-filled airway.

Assume that, in the lung, we wish to explore the motion of a bubble (of volume $V_L = 8 \times 10^6$ μm^3) through a vertical airway of diameter $D_L = 100$ μm. The fluid filling this airway has a density (ρ_L) that is the same as that of water, a viscosity (μ_L) ten times that of water, and a surface tension (σ_L), with respect to air, that is a quarter that of water (72 dyne/cm). The gravitational constant is g in both systems.

(a)   We wish to build an experimental model that is dynamically similar to the situation in the lung. An air bubble (of volume V_m) will be placed into a vertical fluid-filled tube of diameter 0.4 mm. Determine the bubble volume and a set of liquid characteristics such that dynamic similarity is achieved. If there is any flexibility in design requirements, pick characteristics as similar to those of water as possible (to make the experimental design easier to implement).

(b)   Assume that, for this set of experimental conditions, the bubble velocity in the experimental model is measured to be 1 mm/s. Use this information to predict the velocity of the bubble of interest in the lung.

(c)   In the model experiment, a laser was used to measure the gap between the bubble and the tube wall. The closest approach of the bubble to the wall was a distance of 50 μm. Using the experimental results, roughly estimate what the peak shear stress on the lung epithelium would be in an airway of diameter $D_L = 100$ μm through which a bubble of bubble volume $V_L = 8 \times 10^6$ μm^3 was passing. (In making your estimate, you may assume that the bubble behaves like a rigid body.)

9.10. In the airways of the lung, fluid lines the airway walls. This layer of fluid is normally very thin and protects the cells from drying out. However, in diseased states, this layer can become much thicker, filling up a substantial portion of the airway (see the figure at the top of the next page). In this problem, we assume that all of the airways have a fluid lining that is 20% of each airway's radius. You may ignore any influence of breathing in this problem.

Consider the deeper airways of the lung, with radii between 150 and 300 μm. Let the fluid lining these airways have a viscosity of $\mu = 0.02$ g/cm per s, a density of $\rho = 1$ g/cm^3, and a surface tension with respect to air of $\sigma = 25$ g/s^2.

Owing to an instability caused by surface tension, this fluid can flow axially along the airway and accumulate, leading to closure of the airway. We are interested in determining in which airways this process occurs most rapidly.

Determine whether this process proceeds more rapidly in airways with a radius of 150 μm or in those with a diameter of 300 μm, and how much more rapidly it occurs in one than it does in the other. Gravitational effects can be neglected.

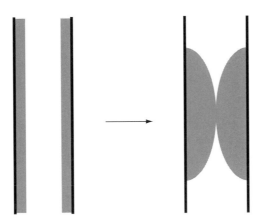

9.11. The viscosity of the cytoplasm of a cell, μ_c, can be determined by pulling a portion of a cell into a micropipette of radius R_m (see the figure below) and measuring the velocity v of the cytoplasm entering the micropipette. The cell is pulled into the micropipette by a pressure drop ΔP across the cell. The radius of the cell is R_c and its density is ρ_c.

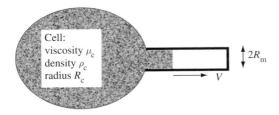

We are interested in predicting how several experimental procedures will affect the steady-state value of v. A baseline study has already been conducted to determine v. For each of the cases below, determine whether a prediction can be made (for the information already available) for the following experimental changes, and, if so, predict (quantitatively) how v will change.

(a) Cutting the pressure drop (ΔP) in half.
(b) Using a smaller micropipette tip with a radius half that used in the baseline case.
(c) Adding an enzyme to the cell such that its viscosity is halved.

It is realized that another property of the cell affects the velocity of aspiration, namely the cell's ability to resist solid deformation, characterized by Young's modulus of elasticity of the cell, E_c. A typical value of E_c for a cell would be 500 Pa. How would this change your answers to parts (a)–(c)?

9.12. When leukocytes adhere to the endothelium of a blood vessel, they undergo an interesting rolling motion. This is caused by the flow of blood over the leukocyte and the force (F) binding the leukocyte to the endothelium. We would like to determine this force.

Consider a blood vessel of radius $R = 100$ μm with a flow of blood ($Q = 0.2 \times 10^{-4}$ cm³/s) passing through the vessel. When viewed under a microscope, a leukocyte of radius 5 μm is seen to be rolling along the wall at a rotational velocity of $\omega = 0.05$ revolutions/s (0.314 radians/s). The density of the blood is 1.05 g/cm³ and its viscosity is 0.04 g/cm per s.

We wish to build a model system that would allow us to determine what the binding force of a leukocyte to the endothelium might be. We will look at the rolling of a latex microsphere along the wall of a round tube (of radius R_m). This microsphere will be made to adhere to the wall of the round tube with a known force F_m.

(a) Derive a set of dimensionless variables for relating the angular velocity of rolling to the other variables.

(b) We have available microspheres of radius 20 μm, each of which will adhere to a plastic substrate with a force (F_m) of 10^{-6} dynes. We also have available a fluid with exactly the same density and viscosity as those of blood. We plan to run a series of experiments in a plastic tube of radius R_m to determine how the rolling rate of the microsphere varies with the flow rate (Q_m). Determine what constraints, if any, need to be put on these experimental variables.

(c) In the model experiment, we find that, for the range of flow rates investigated, ω_m varies with Q_m as

$$\omega_m = \omega_0 + \alpha Q_m$$

where $\omega_0 = 0.001$ revolutions/s ($2\pi \times 10^{-3}$ rad/s) and $\alpha = 10$ revolutions/cm³ (20π rad/cm³).

Assuming that the microsphere and the leukocyte are caused to rotate by the same mechanism, determine the force (F) that makes the leukocyte adhere to the vessel wall.

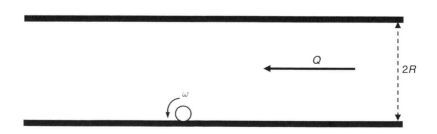

10 Statistical mechanics

(8 problems)

10.1. Nanoparticles can be used to probe the intracellular environment. By tracking their motion one can draw conclusions regarding transport inside a cell.

An investigator has placed a nanoparticle of diameter 100 nm inside of a *Xenopus* oocyte. The cytoplasm of this cell behaves like a viscous fluid with a viscosity 20 times that of water. Over a period of 20 s (at a temperature of 18 °C), the particle travels (on a somewhat erratic path) over a distance of approximately 3 μm from the periphery of the cell toward the nucleus in the center of the cell.

The investigator concludes that there is a preferential motion or "flow" from the periphery of the cell toward the nucleus. He would now like to plan a full study to examine what causes this "flow." Does this seem like a reasonable next step? If so, justify why. If not, explain what next step you would suggest.

10.2. Fibrinogen has a diffusion coefficient in saline of approximately 2×10^{-7} cm^2/s at 25 °C. It is a rod-shaped molecule whose length is roughly 10 times its radius. Estimate the length of this molecule.

10.3. A virus with a molecular weight of 40 million daltons, a density of 1.3 g/ml, and a diffusion coefficient in saline of 3×10^{-8} cm^2/s (at 25 °C) has been discovered. What can you determine about the shape of this virus?

10.4. Hyaluronic acid is a long-chain polyelectrolyte that comes in a variety of molecular weights. Consider a particular fraction whose molecular weight we would like to determine.

The diffusion coefficient of these macromolecules in physiological saline is measured to be 1×10^{-7} cm^2/s. A solution of these macromolecules is put into an ultracentrifuge that spins them at 200 000**g**, in which case they move through saline at a sedimentation velocity of 0.4 cm/h. The density of hyaluronic acid is 1.5 g/ml. All of the measurements mentioned above were made at 25 °C.

Find the molecular weight of this fraction of hyaluronic acid. Derive any needed formulas used that you have not already been given in class.

10.5. If round particles are made from polystyrene (of density 1.05 g/ml), estimate how small they must be in order that they do not sediment out of suspension when placed into water in a 1-cm-tall tube at 25 °C.

10.6. This problem concerns the distribution of air molecules in the atmosphere.

(a) Assuming that the atmosphere is isothermal, find the density of air (n, the number of molecules per unit volume) as a function of height in the atmosphere. (Hint: if gravity is always pulling air molecules downward, what force is keeping them up?)

(b) Now, consider a different view of this process, with the air molecules falling downward at a terminal velocity V, but also diffusing upward due to a concentration gradient with a diffusion coefficient D. Using the results from part (a), find a relationship between V and D.

(c) By treating an air molecule as a sphere of radius R and mass m, find the terminal velocity V that a falling air molecule will have if it is acted on by gravity and moves through a fluid (air) that has a viscosity of μ. Use this result to find the diffusion coefficient of air. The resulting equation is known as the Stokes–Einstein equation.

10.7. Linear macromolecules in solution are sometimes modeled as a collection of massless balls connected by frictionless springs. The hydrodynamic behavior of the macromolecule is then described by balancing the spring forces acting on these balls with the frictional forces that act on the moving balls.

Consider a simple model of such a macromolecule consisting of two balls and a single spring connecting them. Each ball has a radius of $R = 5$ nm. The spring force can be found as $F = \gamma(x - x_0)$, where x is the distance between the centers of the two balls, $x_0 = 20$ nm and $\gamma = k_B T / x_0^2$, where k_B is Boltzmann's constant and T is the absolute temperature.

(a) If this molecule is placed into water at 25 °C, and then is stretched such that $x - x_0 = 0.5x_0$, and released, calculate the time constant for this molecule to return to its undeformed state (i.e. τ such that $x(\tau) - x_0 = [x(t=0) - x_0] e^{-1}$). This is known as the Zimm time.

(b) If this molecule is placed into a shear flow, and left there for a time long compared with the Zimm time, what will the final orientation of the molecule relative to the direction of flow be? Use the spring-and-balls model to explain your answer.

10.8. The Langevin equation describes the Brownian motion of a particle (of mass m_p) allowing for random forces that are due to molecular collisions. The forces acting on a particle include the viscous force which is proportional to the particle velocity (Stokes' law) and a noise term accounting for the other molecular collisions. In the x-direction, this equation is written as

$$m_p \frac{dv_x}{dt} = -f v_x + F'(t)$$

where f is the frictional coefficient from Stokes' law and F' is a random force that has the following characteristics:

$$\langle F'(t) \rangle = 0$$

and

$$\langle F'(t) x(t) \rangle = 0$$

Furthermore,

$$m_p \left\langle \frac{v_x^2}{2} \right\rangle = \frac{k_B T}{2}$$

The angle brackets, $\langle \ \rangle$, denote the ensemble average (an average over all particles at a particular instant in time). The first condition just indicates that there is no mean force except for the Stokes force, which acts opposite to the direction of motion. The second condition is that the force is random and uncorrelated with the particle position. The final condition expresses the equipartition of energy: each degree of freedom (in this case, just the x-direction) has the same energy, which is that specified by Boltzmann's constant, k_B).

(a) Show that the Langevin equation can be written in the following form:

$$\frac{m_p}{2} \frac{d^2 \langle x^2 \rangle}{dt^2} - k_B T + \frac{f}{2} \frac{d \langle x^2 \rangle}{dt} = 0.$$

(b) Show that a solution to this equation is

$$\langle x^2(t) \rangle = \frac{2 k_B T}{f} t - \frac{2 m_p k_B T}{f^2} \left[1 - \exp\left(-\frac{ft}{m_p} \right) \right]$$

   if $\langle x^2 \rangle$ and $d \langle x^2 \rangle / dt$ both equal zero at $t = 0$.

(c) Using the binomial expansion of $\exp(-y)$ with $y \ll 1$, show that the short-time behavior described by the equation from part (b) predicts "ballistic" behaviour ($\langle x^2 \rangle \sim t^2$) for short times ($t \ll m_p/f$). Similarly, show that it predicts diffusive behavior ($\langle x^2 \rangle \sim t$) for long times, and find the corresponding diffusion coefficient.

11 Steady diffusion and conduction

(17 diffusion problems; 3 conduction problems)

11.1. Consider a tissue surrounded on both sides by a fluid. A species S is diffusing across this tissue, and has concentrations C_1^F and C_2^F (in the fluid) on the two sides of the tissue, as shown in the figure below. The solubility of species S inside the tissue is different from its solubility in the fluid. We therefore define a partition coefficient Φ:

$$\Phi = C_1^T/C_1^F = C_2^T/C_2^F$$

where C_1^T and C_2^T are concentrations of species S in the tissue at faces 1 and 2 of the tissue, respectively.

Hence $\Phi < 1$ means that S is less soluble in the tissue, and vice versa. Write down an expression for the mass-transfer rate per unit area across the tissue in terms of C_1^F, C_2^F, D_T (the diffusion coefficient of S in the tissue), Δy, and Φ.

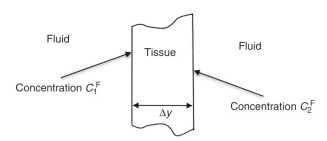

11.2. We are interested in comparing the steady-state CO_2 concentrations in two cell-culture systems. Assume that each cell produces m moles of CO_2 per second, a constant under all culture conditions. The diffusion coefficient of the CO_2 in saline is D.

(a) Assume that N cells are plated to the bottom of a tissue culture dish (see the figure below) of area A, and that these cells are covered with saline to a depth δ. Air is constantly circulated over the saline such that the CO_2 concentration is essentially zero at the surface of the saline. Find the maximum CO_2 concentration in the saline. (The height of the cells is negligible compared with δ.)

(b) Now assume that these N cells are instead uniformly distributed in the saline (see the figure) in this tissue culture dish under the same conditions as in part (a). Find the maximum CO_2 concentration in the saline.

(Hint: in part (a) CO_2 is generated only at the base of the dish, whereas in part (b) the generation of CO_2 occurs homogeneously everywhere in the fluid.)

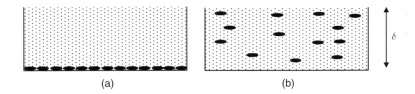

(a)   (b)

11.3. Consider the diffusion of a drug from a cylindrical disk. For a thin disk (of thickness $H \ll S$, where S is the radius), diffusion from the disk into the surrounding tissues can be treated as a one-dimensional problem in the direction along the axis of the disk.

(a) A drug is being released uniformly from the material contained in the disk at a fixed rate $\dot{\varepsilon}$ (moles per unit volume per unit time). Find an expression for the steady-state concentration profile of the drug inside the disk. You may assume that the drug diffuses so freely in the surrounding tissue, relative to within the disk, that the surface concentrations, $C(x = 0)$ and $C(x = H)$, can both be assumed to be zero.

(b) Compute the steady flux (moles per unit time) of drug out of the disk at $x = 0$ and $x = H$.

11.4. Consider the same figure as for Problem 11.2. We are interested in examining the effects of low concentrations of nitrous oxide (N_2O) on cell behavior in two cell-culture systems. In each case, cells are in culture medium in a dish, but in the first situation the cells are at the bottom of the dish, whereas in at the second they are uniformly distributed in the medium.

The surface of the liquid is held at an N_2O concentration of C_0 (g/ml) by mass exchange with the gas above the media. The concentration of gas in the liquid below the surface is $C(x)$, where $0 < x < \delta$.

Assume that a cell at a location x takes up N_2O at a rate of

$$\dot{\varepsilon} = -KC(x)$$

where $\dot{\varepsilon}$ has units of g/s. K is a constant everywhere in the system. The diffusion coefficient of the N_2O in the culture medium is D. Assume steady-state conditions.

(a) First consider the situation when N cells are plated to the bottom of a tissue culture dish (see the figure for Problem 11.2) of area A, and these cells are covered with culture medium to a depth δ. Find the minimum concentration of N_2O in the culture medium. (The height of the cells is negligible compared with δ.)

(b) Now assume that these N cells are instead uniformly distributed in the culture medium (see the figure for Problem 11.2) in this tissue culture dish under the same conditions as in part (a). Find the minimum concentration of N_2O in the culture medium.

(Hint: in part (a) the consumption of N_2O occurs only at the base of the dish, whereas in part (b) the consumption of N_2O occurs homogeneously everywhere in the fluid.)

11.5. Small porous particles can be used for sustained drug delivery. One such system uses particles approximately 1 mm in diameter that are impregnated with the drug to be delivered. Drug delivery continues for a two-week period. During the first several days of drug delivery, the drug-release rate from the particles is essentially constant everywhere at 0.1×10^{-9} mol/s per cm^3.

The diffusion coefficient of the drug within the particle is 1×10^{-8} cm^2/s while the diffusion coefficient of the drug in the tissue in which the particle is placed is 1×10^{-6} cm^2/s. You may ignore any uptake of the drug by cells in the tissue, and binding of the drug to the tissue. The tissue of interest is avascular. Thus, the drug is transported solely by diffusion.

Consider a SINGLE particle placed into a much, much larger tissue. A few hours after the particle has been placed in the tissue, assume that the drug being released from the particle has reached a quasi-steady-state concentration distribution in the tissue surrounding the particle. After this quasi-steady-state has been reached, find

(a) the total rate of drug delivery from the particle to the tissue and

(b) the concentration of drug in the tissue immediately adjacent to the surface of the particle.

11.6. From an oxygen-consumption point of view, the retina can be considered to be made up of four layers:

(1) the outer segments (length $L_1 = 35$ µm);
(2) the inner segments, rich in oxygen-using mitochondria (length $L_2 = 30$ µm);
(3) the outer nuclear layer (length $L_3 = 55$ µm); and
(4) the rest of the retina (not considered in this model; it contains retinal blood vessels and oxygen-consuming tissue).

Oxygen is consumed only in layers 2 and 4. Assume that the oxygen-consumption rate per unit volume of tissue is $e = 3 \times 10^{-5}$ g/cm^3 per s. Let the oxygen diffusivity be $D = 2 \times 10^{-5}$ cm^2/s, and assume it to be the same in all layers; you may also assume that the partition coefficient of oxygen in all tissues is 1.

If oxygen is provided at a concentration $C_0 = 1.8 \times 10^{-5}$ g/cm^3 at the outer surface of layer 1 ($x = 0$) and at $C_4 = 0.6 \times 10^{-5}$ g/cm^3 at the inner surface of layer 3 ($x = L_1 + L_2 + L_3$), find the minimum oxygen level in the retina. In the figure, the dark line shows qualitatively what the oxygen concentration profile, $C(x)$, should look like.

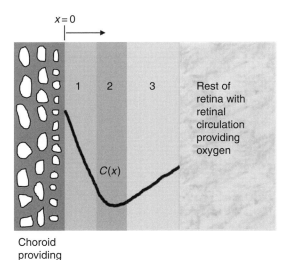

11.7. Consider a growth factor (e.g. KGF) that is released into the extravascular space such that its concentration C_0 in the extracellular space is constant and equal to 1 µM. The goal is to deliver the KGF to the endothelium of a blood vessel passing through this space.

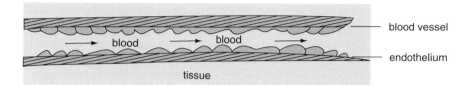

The outer radius of the vessel (R_o) is 200 μm and the inner radius (R_i) is 150 μm. The thickness of the endothelial lining is 1 μm. The diffusion coefficient of the KGF passing through the vessel wall is 1×10^{-7} cm^2/s, while the diffusion coefficient of the KGF passing through the endothelium is 1×10^{-9} cm^2/s. You may assume that the concentration of KGF in flowing blood is essentially zero.

Find the average concentration of KGF in the endothelial lining assuming steady-state conditions. (Hint: remember that the endothelial lining is very thin; the picture is not to scale.)

11.8. In one design for a bioreactor, a mixture of cells and extracellular matrix is cast into the shape of long, cylindrical fibers. The fibers are placed into a tank in which fluid is flowing. The cells produce a cytokine that can then be collected as it diffuses out of the fibers and into the flowing stream. However, this cytokine is toxic to the cells at high concentration, and thus we must ensure that, everywhere within the fibers, the concentration of this cytokine does not become too high. The maximum safe concentration is 1×10^{-5} mol/cm^3.

The cells produce this cytokine at a rate of $S = 0.3 \times 10^{-7}$ mol/s per cm^3 of fiber. Let the mass-transfer coefficient characterizing the flux ($j_{surface}$) of cytokine at the fiber surface be determined by $j_{surface} = h_m C(r = R)$, where R is the fiber radius and $h_m = 2 \times 10^{-5}$ cm/s. The diffusion coefficient for the cytokine within the fibers is $D = 5 \times 10^{-5}$ cm^2/s. The fibers have a radius of $R = 0.1$ cm and a length of $L = 2$ cm.

(a) What is the appropriate mass transfer boundary condition at the surface of the fiber?

(b) Determine whether or not the maximum safe concentration of cytokine will be exceeded anywhere within the fiber.

(c) What is the total rate at which cytokine leaves the fiber?

11.9. One of the challenges of making artificial tissue constructs is the need to provide adequate oxygen to the cells in thick tissue regions before the construct is vascularized. One possible solution is to implant tiny spheres of radius 100 μm into the construct. These spheres release oxygen through a chemical reaction. We want oxygen to be delivered at a rate such that cells are kept viable out to a distance of 200 μm from the center of the sphere (but no further).

Consider a single sphere surrounded by tissue and ignore the influence of other spheres. Assume steady-state conditions, that the tissue has an oxygen-consumption rate (per unit volume) of $s = 3 \times 10^{-6}$ g/cm^3 per s, and that the diffusion constant for the passage of oxygen through the tissue is 1.7×10^{-5} cm^2/s.

(a)   Assuming that the cells are not viable at radii greater than 200 μm from the center of a sphere, what is the concentration of oxygen at $r = 200$ μm, and what is the total oxygen flux passing that location?

(b)   What would be the total rate of oxygen transfer (g/s) from the surface of each sphere necessary in order to keep the cells viable out to a distance of 200 μm from the center of the sphere (but no further)?

(c)   It is important to make sure that the concentration of oxygen is not too high in the tissue so as to avoid toxicity to the cells. Assuming that the oxygen flux provided to the tissue (J_{O_2}) is equal to that determined in part (b), what would be the maximum concentration of oxygen within the tissue surrounding one of these spheres, and where would this maximum concentration occur?

11.10. The figure [11] overleaf shows the effects of occluding an artery in the cerebellum of the opossum by a spore (arrow). Capillaries in the cerebellum are the elongated structures distributed throughout the tissue, one of which is occluded by the spore. The small nerve cells have died in a 25-μm region surrounding the blocked capillaries. The nerve cells around the neighboring functional capillaries are intact.

Capillary beds can be modeled as repeating structures in which the basic unit is a single capillary surrounded by a cylindrical tissue region. We wish to determine the maximum cylinder size such that all of the tissue in the cylinder receives an adequate oxygen supply. This cylinder is known as the Krogh cylinder. Any tissue outside of this cylinder does not receive any oxygen (from this capillary).

Consider a capillary of radius 5 μm that carries blood with an oxygen tension of 95 mm Hg (the partial pressure which is equivalent to the concentration of oxygen in the tissue). Let the tissue surrounding this capillary have an oxygen-consumption rate (per unit volume) of 180 mm Hg/s and let the diffusion constant of oxygen through tissue be 1.7×10^{-5} cm^2/s. Find the radius at which the tissue would become anoxic, assuming that there is no transfer of oxygen from any neighboring capillaries. (Hint: what are the boundary conditions at the anoxic border?)

You may assume that the diffusion coefficient for the passage of oxygen across the endothelial cell layer lining the capillary is comparable to that in the surrounding tissue. The difference between the (greater) oxygen-consumption rate of the endothelial cell layer and that of the surrounding tissue can be neglected.

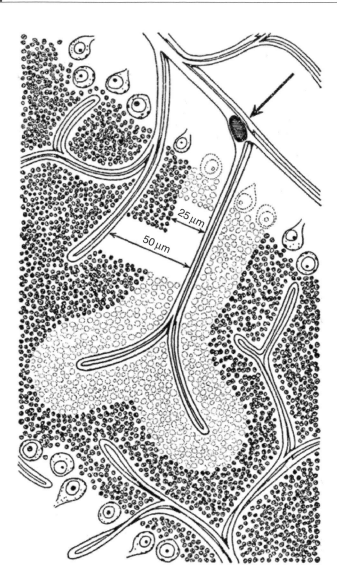

11.11. When tumors grow, they become vascularized so that the tumor cells can get adequate oxygen. We are interested in how large a tumor can become without having its own blood supply. Consider a spherical, avascular tumor of radius R under steady-state conditions. We would like to find how large R can become while still having the tumor receive an adequate oxygen supply.

The tumor tissue consumes oxygen at a rate (per unit volume) of 10^{-5} g/cm^3 per s. Let the diffusivity of oxygen in the tumor be 2×10^{-5} cm^2/s. The tissue surrounding the tumor has an oxygen tension of 1.7×10^{-5} g/cm^3. Consider two possible boundary conditions at the surface of the tumor.

(a) Let the concentration of oxygen at the surface of the tumor be the same as that in the surrounding tissue (1.7×10^{-5} g/cm^3). For this boundary condition, find the maximum radius (R) of the tumor such that all of the tumor cells receive an adequate oxygen supply.

(b) Let the flux of oxygen that is supplied to the tumor by blood in the tissue surrounding the tumor be $j = 8.5 \times 10^{-8}$ g/cm^2 per s. For this boundary condition, find the maximum radius (R) of the tumor such that all of the tumor cells receive an adequate oxygen supply.

11.12. Cells are increasingly used as biochemical factories to make a variety of bioactive agents. One design for use of these cells is to incorporate them into long cylindrical polymeric rods. These rods are highly porous, and thus allow oxygen and nutrient exchange with the cells.

Consider such cylindrical rods that are each 25 μm in radius and 4 mm long. Cells are incorporated uniformly into these cylinders, and these cells then produce a desired peptide. We are concerned that the cells receive an adequate oxygen supply.

Let the oxygen tension at the surface of each cylinder be constant at 2.8×10^{-6} g/ml. Assume a diffusion coefficient for oxygen through the porous cell-filled rods of 1×10^{-5} cm^2/s. Let the oxygen-consumption rate within the rods be 1.1×10^{-5} g/ml per s per unit volume of rod. Will all the cells inside the rods receive an adequate amount of oxygen?

11.13. A sphere of radius $R_0 = 0.1$ cm made of a soluble polymer is placed into a very large solution of stationary fluid in which the polymer begins to dissolve. You may assume that this process occurs slowly enough that the concentration of polymer everywhere in the solution is quasi-steady (there is no time-dependence, except for $R(t)$). The concentration of polymer is to be assumed always constant inside the sphere and equal to $C_0 = 10$ mg/ml. The diffusion coefficient of the polymer in the fluid is 1×10^{-6} cm^2/s. For the quasi-steady situation considered here, the concentration of polymer in the fluid immediately adjacent to the sphere can be considered to be constant with a value of $C_s = 1$ mg/ml. How long will it take for the sphere to dissolve?

11.14. In an air-filled room in a space station in orbit, a droplet of CCl$_4$ (of radius 2 mm) is released. The total pressure in the room is 760 mm Hg (at $T = 0$ °C), and the vapor pressure of the CCl$_4$ is 33 mm Hg. The diffusivity of the CCl_4 in air is approximately 0.065 cm^2/s. Assume that the air is essentially insoluble in the CCl_4. Note that the concentration of CCl_4 in air cannot be considered dilute.

(a)   Assuming a quasi-static radius of the droplet, find the steady-state concentration distribution of air around the droplet, $C_a(r)$.

(b)   How long will it take for the droplet to evaporate? Let the density of liquid CCl_4 be 1.59 g/ml, and let its molecular weight be 154.

11.15. Chemotaxis is a process by which a cell moves toward a chemical signal. It is thought that the cell senses the gradient in the concentration of a chemical and then moves toward the higher concentration. However, it could be that a different mechanism is involved. It has been hypothesized that cells can alter their random motions (i.e. their diffusion coefficient) as a function of the local concentration of the chemoattractant.

To evaluate this assumption, consider the following model system (a Boyden chamber) in which the cells are introduced on one side of a porous medium ($x = 0$) and collected by a filter on the other side (at $x = L$). The concentration of cells at $x = 0$ is $C_c = C_0$, and this concentration can be considered constant. Because the cells captured at $x = L$ by the filter can no longer diffuse, the concentration of cells at $x = L$ can be taken as $C_c = 0$. The chemoattractant is released from $x = L$ with concentration α, and is removed at $x = 0$, and thus its concentration there is 0. Its diffusion coefficient is D_a, which is constant everywhere. Let the diffusion coefficient of the cells in the porous medium depend on the local concentration of the chemoattractant as

$$D_c(x) = D_0[1 + pC_a(x)]$$

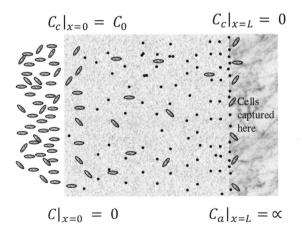

$$C_c|_{x=0} = C_0 \qquad C_c|_{x=L} = 0$$

$$C|_{x=0} = 0 \qquad C_a|_{x=L} = \alpha$$

Assume steady-state conditions.

(a) Evaluate the hypothesis that chemoattraction can result from cells increasing (or decreasing) their diffusion coefficient in response to an increase (or decrease) in the local concentration of the chemoattractant. Explain why this hypothesis might be correct, or must be false.

(b) If you concluded that the hypothesis is valid, solve for the flux of cells into the filter as a function of p and α. If you concluded that it is false, show that the flux of cells into the filter is independent of p and α.

11.16. Consider the transport of oxygen in **stagnant** blood. More specifically, suppose that a large container filled with deoxygenated whole blood is suddenly placed in an atmosphere of pure oxygen. The concentration of unbound oxygen at the surface of the blood (in solution) is C_0, where C_0 is constant. Because of the very nonlinear nature with which hemoglobin binds oxygen, this leads to the formation and propagation of a "front." Above this interface the hemoglobin is oxygenated and there is free (unbound) oxygen in solution in the plasma, while below this interface the free-oxygen concentration is zero and the hemoglobin is deoxygenated. The front location, z_f, advances slowly with time.

(a) Find the oxygen concentration profile above the interface and show that the flux of oxygen into the blood, n, is given by

$$n = DC_0/z_f$$

where D is the diffusivity of oxygen in whole blood and z_f is the position of the front. For the purposes of this portion of the question, you may assume that the front is slowly moving, compared with the time-scale for diffusion. State other assumptions.

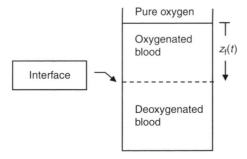

(b) Assuming that four moles of oxygen will bind rapidly and irreversibly to one mole of hemoglobin at the front, and that the concentration of deoxygenated hemoglobin below the front is C_{Hb}, find $z_f(t)$. Note that $C_{Hb} \gg C_0$.
(Hint: perform an unsteady mass balance on the oxygen in the container. Don't forget to take into account oxygen that is bound irreversibly to hemoglobin.) From [2].

11.17. In recent experiments, it has been shown that a particular type of peptide-based gel, when injected into the myocardium, elicits an angiogenic response, with the ingrowth of vessels and invasion by neighboring myocytes into the gel. Here we consider just the first stage of this process, namely the equilibration of the gel implant with the concentrations of growth factors in the surrounding tissue.

To simplify, consider the diffusion of solute from surrounding tissue into a spherical implant of radius a. The solute of interest binds to the gel irreversibly according to first-order kinetics with rate constant k. You may assume that the concentration of the solute at the surface of the sphere is approximately constant, C_0, and that the diffusion coefficient, D, is known.

(a) Write the governing equation for transport within the spherical gel and specify the boundary conditions. You should assume that diffusion occurs rapidly compared with the time over which the concentration changes due to chemical reaction; that is, the concentration distribution is quasi-steady at all times, and the unsteady term can be neglected.
(b) Introduce a dimensionless radius, $\eta = r/a$, and concentration, $C^* = C/C_0$, and show that the behavior of the solution is governed by a single dimensionless group:

$$\varphi = a(k/D)^{1/2}$$

This group is called the Thiele modulus and represents the ratio of the diffusion time to the reaction time. (Note that this is similar in form to the Damköhler number, which represents the ratio of the *transport* time to the reaction time. If transport is by diffusion alone, then the two take the same form.)
(c) Solve this equation, using the hint that you should look for a solution using the substitute variable $\theta = C^* \eta$. Plot the concentration distribution, C^*, as a function of η for several values of the Thiele modulus ($\varphi = 1.0$, 10, and 100).

11.18. A solid cylinder of radius R and length L is made from material with thermal conductivity k. Heat is generated inside the cylinder at a rate S (energy per unit volume per unit time).

(a) Neglecting conduction along the axis of the cylinder, find the steady-state temperature distribution in the cylinder, given that the surface temperature is T_s.

(b) Consider a crude approximation of a mouse modeled as a cylinder of radius 1 cm and length 5 cm. If the ambient air temperature is 10 °C and the internal rate of heat generation in the animal is 10^{-3} W/cm^3, find the skin temperature (T_s) for the mouse. The external heat-transfer coefficient is $h = 0.2$ W/m^2 per K.

11.19. Elephants, due to their low ratio of surface area to tissue volume, have difficulties with removal of heat from their bodies. Their large ears greatly aid in this process. We would like to model their ears as fins and determine the amount of heat they can remove from their bodies by flapping their ears. You may assume steady-state conditions.

(a) We first want to derive a differential equation that describes the temperature of their ears as a function of the radial distance (r) from the center of the ear (we will model the ear as a half-disk). The radius of the elephant ear is approximately 60 cm, and its thickness is 1 cm. Heat is lost from the ears as they flap, and the heat-transfer coefficient at the surface of the ear is h. The temperature surrounding the ear is T_∞.

Unlike in the standard analysis of heat transfer from a fin, we must take into account that blood is delivering heat to the tissue. The net transfer of energy (per unit tissue volume) can be written as $s = \omega \rho c (T_a - T(r))$, where ω is the rate of blood perfusion to the tissue (volume of blood per unit tissue volume per unit time), ρ is the density of the blood, c is its heat capacity, T_a is the temperature of the arterial blood, and $T(r)$ is the temperature of the tissue (we are here assuming that the venous blood leaving the tissue has the same temperature as does the tissue).

Derive a differential equation that describes the radial temperature distribution in the flapping elephant ear. Let k represent the thermal conductivity of the tissue. You can neglect any heat generation by the ear tissues themselves.

(b) Now assume that conduction of heat from one location to another in the ear is insignificant. Let $\omega = 0.005$ s^{-1}, $\rho = 1$ g/cm^3, $c = 4200$ J/kg per °C, $k = 0.6$ W/m per °C, $T_a = 37$ °C, $T_\infty = 25$ °C, and $h = 20$ W/m^2 per °C. Find the temperature distribution, $T(r)$, of the elephant ear.

(c) Evaluate whether the assumption that heat conduction can be neglected is reasonable.

11.20. The rat's tail is well suited to function as a heat-loss organ. It lacks fur, has a large surface-area-to-volume ratio, and is well vascularized with arteriovenous anastomoses. We first want to derive a differential equation that describes the temperature of the rat tail as a function of distance from the rat's hind end. Take the length of the rat tail to be approximately 15 cm (this is a New York City rat) and its diameter to be 4 mm. The heat-transfer coefficient at the surface of the tail is h, and the air temperature surrounding the tail is T_∞. You may assume steady-state conditions.

Unlike in the standard analysis of heat transfer from a fin, we must take into account that the blood is delivering heat to the tissue. The net transfer of energy (per unit tissue volume) can be written as $s = \omega\rho c(T_a - T)$, where ω is the rate of blood perfusion to the tissue (the volume of blood per unit tissue volume per unit time), ρ is the density of the blood, c is its heat capacity, T_a is the temperature of the arterial blood, and T is the temperature of the tissue (we are here assuming that the venous blood leaving the tissue has the same temperature as does the tissue).

(a) Derive a differential equation that describes the axial temperature distribution in the rat tail. Let k represent the thermal conductivity of the tissue. You can neglect any heat generation by the tail tissues themselves.

(b) Now assume that conduction of heat from one location to another in the tail is insignificant. Let $\omega = 0.01$ s^{-1}, $\rho = 1$ g/cm^3, $c = 4200$ J/kg per °C, $k = 0.6$ W/m per °C, $T_a = 37$ °C, $T_\infty = 25$ °C, and $h = 5$ W/m^2 per °C. Find the temperature distribution, $T(x)$, as a function of distance along the rat tail.

(c) Evaluate whether the assumption that heat conduction can be neglected is reasonable.

12 Unsteady diffusion and conduction

(21 unsteady diffusion; 3 unsteady conduction)

12.1. We want to determine how fast the alveolar CO_2 concentration can change in response to changes in blood CO_2 concentration. Assume a spherically shaped alveolus (of radius 0.015 cm) with a spatially uniform internal gaseous composition at time $t = 0$. Calculate the time necessary to achieve 95% equilibration when the CO_2 concentration in the alveolar wall is suddenly changed at $t = 0$. You may neglect any mass-transfer effects of the wall tissue and the liquid film in the alveolus. The diffusion coefficient of CO_2 in air is 0.14 cm^2/s.

Considering your answer, how important is the diffusion resistance to mass transport through the gas contained within the alveolus?

12.2. Fluorescein is a small fluorescent tracer molecule that is used in a wide variety of physiologic studies. In the eye, it is used in a technique known as fluorophotometry to characterize the transport characteristics of aqueous humor, the fluid that fills the anterior chamber behind the cornea.

A drop of fluorescein (50 μl of 0.005%, by mass, fluorescein in saline) is placed onto the cornea and spreads evenly over the corneal surface to create a thin film. It then diffuses through the cornea ($D = 1 \times 10^{-6}$ cm^2/s) and enters the aqueous humor on the back side of the cornea. The thickness of the cornea is about 0.05 cm and its radius is 0.5 cm.

(a) Estimate how much fluorescein will enter the cornea during the first minute after application.
(b) Estimate how long it will take before a detectable quantity of fluorescein (0.0001%) begins to enter the aqueous humor.

12.3. A drug manufacturer is designing a round pellet (1 mm in diameter) to slowly release a large therapeutic macromolecule into connective tissues. Connective tissues are filled with a fibrous extracellular matrix and the interfiber spacing through which the drug needs to diffuse is similar in size to that of the macromolecule to be delivered to the tissue. This is advantageous for delivery of the drug insofar as it will slow the release process and allow the drug to be released over a longer time period. The pellet is designed such that it is similar in physical structure to the extracellular matrix, which facilitates the slow release of the drug.

Two important issues in the design of this pellet are (i) what the diffusion coefficient of this drug in the extracellular matrix will be and (ii) how much drug is loaded into each pellet. The answers to both of these questions are important for use in calculations on drug kinetics.

To answer these two questions, the manufacturer placed the pellet in a large chamber (10 cm in diameter) filled with a fibrous extracellular matrix that models the tissue in which the pellet will be placed. The concentration of drug is then measured optically as a function of time at a location 0.5 cm away from the center of the pellet. The peak drug concentration was found to occur 95 hours after the pellet had been placed in the matrix, and the peak concentration of drug at that location (0.5 cm from the center of the pellet) was found to be 1 μg/ml.

Since the pellet is similar in composition to the extracellular matrix, and the pellet is very small, the drug can be assumed to be a depot placed at a point and to have the same diffusion coefficient everywhere in the chamber. Find the diffusion coefficient of the macromolecule in the fibrous extracellular matrix, and determine the mass of drug that was loaded into the pellet.

12.4. Porous spheres (400 μm in diameter) are uniformly impregnated with a drug at a concentration of C_0 (1 mg/ml). These spheres are then placed into tissues to allow the slow (quasi-steady) release of this drug into the tissue. Consider one such sphere and assume that the drug concentration far from the sphere is negligible. Assuming a diffusivity of the drug in the porous spheres of $D_s = 1 \times 10^{-10}$ cm^2/s while the diffusivity of the drug in the tissue is $D_t = 10^{-6}$ cm^2/s, estimate when the average concentration of drug in the porous sphere will have dropped to 10% of its original value.

12.5. An experimental system has been designed to examine the transient shape changes of cells in an extracellular matrix when stimulated by a chemical agent. The cells are grown in the matrix in a concentric annular shell (see the figure) that has an inner radius of a and an outer radius of b. Fluid flows inside the tube so that the cells can be exposed to oxygen, nutrients, and experimental agents. There is a filter (represented by the dark, dashed line in the figure) that extends the length of the tube on the inside of the concentric shell that keeps the matrix and cells inside.

The shape of the cells is determined by rapidly introducing fixative into the system and then looking at the cells under a microscope. We want to see how quickly the cells can be fixed.

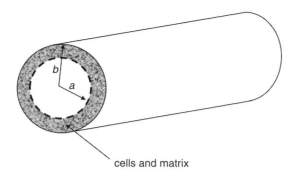

cells and matrix

Let the fixative be introduced to the system in the flow inside the tube at a concentration of 4 mM. Let the flow inside the tube be rapid enough that the concentration is everywhere constant in the flowing fluid inside the tube as soon as it is introduced inside the tube. This concentration can be assumed to be constant in time. Let the diffusion coefficient of fixative within the cell–matrix layer be $D = 4 \times 10^{-5}$ cm^2/s. Let the mass-transfer coefficient characterizing mass transport of fixative from the flowing fluid across the filter to the matrix and cells be $h_m = 1 \times 10^{-5}$ cm/s. Let the radius b be 0.2 cm and the radius a be 0.19 cm. The length of the tube is $L = 5$ cm.

Find how long it takes for the fixative to pass through the filter into the matrix and cells such that all cells are exposed to a concentration of fixative of at least 3 mM.

12.6. In one experimental form of cancer treatment, an inactive cellular toxin is injected into the vascular system. It permeates the entire body and is then cleared

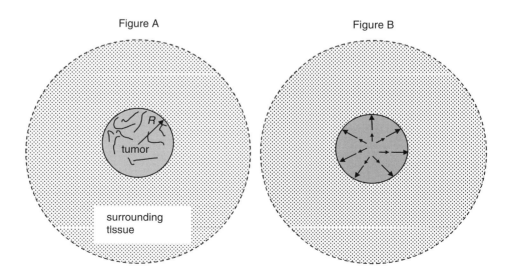

Figure A   Figure B

tumor

surrounding tissue

from the vascular system, but remains in the interstitial space. Then, this toxin is photo-activated only in the region of the tumor, using a laser, killing the tumor cells in that region. Following activation, the toxin is lost from the tumor primarily by reabsorption into the blood, but also by transport to the surrounding tissue. We wish to determine for how long this activated toxin will kill cancer cells, and how much collateral damage might be caused as this activated toxin is then transported to the surrounding tissue.

Assume that the tumor can be modeled as a spherical tissue mass surrounded by normal tissue (see figure A). Tumors are fairly open tissues (compared with the surrounding tissue), and this facilitates transport within the tumor. The diffusion coefficient (D_{tumor}) within the tumor is so high that the concentration of toxin within the tumor can be assumed to be uniform. The dense connective tissue that surrounds the tumor has a much lower diffusion coefficient (D_{tissue}).

The parameters are tumor radius $R = 0.5$ cm, $D_{tumor} = D_1 = 5 \times 10^{-6}$ cm^2/s, and $D_{tissue} = D_0 = 5 \times 10^{-7}$ cm^2/s.

(a) Assume that the rate of reabsorption of activated toxin back into the blood is characterized by $j = kC(r)$ (mass/surface area of blood vessels per unit time), where k is a mass-transport coefficient, $kA = 0.85 \times 10^{-4}$ cm^3/s, $C(r)$ is the local concentration of activated toxin, and A is the surface area of blood vessels (capillaries) in the tumor. Assuming that the toxin is effective until its concentration drops below 10% of its original activated concentration, calculate how long you expect the toxin to be effective at killing cancer cells. (Assume, for this part of the problem only, that the toxin is lost from the tumor only by reabsorption into the blood.)

(b) Estimate how far away from the tumor you expect there to be collateral cellular damage during this period.

(c) The blood vessels in the tumor are very leaky, and this generates a steady-state, radial interstitial flow out of the tumor (see figure B). Assume that the net fluid leakage rate (e, a flow rate per unit volume) in the tumor is 0.05×10^{-5} cm^3/s per cm^3 of tissue. Find the leakage velocity $V(r)$ of the lymph, where r is the distance from the center of the tumor.

(d) Will this interstitial flow alter your estimate from part (a)? Justify your answer numerically.

12.7. A semi-permeable membrane that allows small proteins to pass freely, but blocks the transport of larger proteins, has been developed. We wish to measure the permeability of this membrane to albumin.

This membrane can be made into spherical shells containing protein solutions. Consider such a spherical shell of radius 0.005 cm containing a solution of fluoresceinated albumin in saline. The diffusivity of the albumin in the saline is 8×10^{-8} cm^2/s.

This sphere is placed into a saline solution that is albumin-free. A laser is used to monitor the albumin concentration at the center of the sphere. The albumin is slowly lost from the sphere through the membrane to the surrounding solution. Owing to the large volume of this surrounding solution, it can be assumed to remain albumin-free. The concentration of albumin at the center of the sphere decreases by 50% over a time of 3 h.

Determine the mass-transfer coefficient (h_m) that characterizes albumin transport across this membrane. Justify any assumptions that you make.

12.8. A drug in a saline vehicle (concentration $C_0 = 1$ mg/ml) is delivered to a patient through an intravenous tube. After the desired amount of drug (10 mg) has been delivered, the upstream valve is closed so that the flow stops (see the figure below). However, the intravenous needle is left in the vein of the patient. Determine how much additional drug enters the patient by diffusion during the hour after closure of the valve.

The tube carrying the drug in solution has a length of 20 cm and a diameter of 3 mm. The infusion needle that goes into the patient's arm is 1 cm long and is 25-gauge (i.e. has an inner diameter of 0.241 mm). The diffusivity of the drug is 5×10^{-6} cm^2/s. State any assumptions that you make.

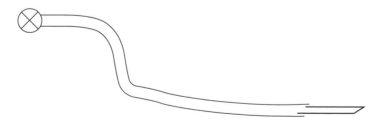

12.9. In a biotech process, biopolymer fibers are made by loading a solution of monomers into porous cylinders (see the figure below), each with an inner radius (R) of 150 μm and a length (L) of 3 mm. The monomers will polymerize into a polymer network inside the porous cylinders when they are exposed to saline at a concentration greater than 100 mM. We will consider the process occurring inside one such porous cylinder.

The porous cylinder, loaded with the monomer solution, is placed into a large water bath. Initially, the bath and porous cylinders are everywhere saline-free. Then, at $t = 0$, the bath fluid is changed such that the solution (outside of the porous cylinders) is everywhere at a saline concentration (C_∞) of 400 mm. The ends of the tube are closed, so saline can enter only by passing through the porous walls of the tube. The diffusion coefficient of saline in the monomer solution is $D = 2 \times 10^{-5}$ cm^2/s. This diffusion rate is unchanged by the polymerization process, and the monomer concentration is sufficiently low that the polymerization reaction has no significant influence on the concentration of salt at any location.

The solution outside the cylinders is rapidly mixed. We denote by h_m the mass-transport coefficient characterizing the flux of salt which is transported across the porous cylinder wall: $j = h_m[C_\infty - C(r = R, t)]$, where $C(r, t)$ is the concentration of salt inside the porous cylinder as a function of the distance r from the center of the cylinder, for $r \le R$.

We wish to find the rate at which the polymer network will form inside the porous cylinders.

(a) Let $h_m = 1 \times 10^{-7}$ cm/s. Determine the time necessary for the polymerization process to be completed inside the cylinder under these conditions.

(b) Now let $h_m = 1$ cm/s. Again, determine the time necessary for the polymerization process to be completed inside the cylinder under these conditions.

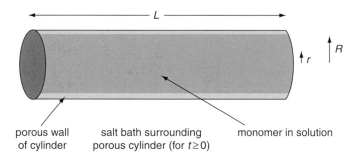

porous wall   salt bath surrounding   monomer in solution
of cylinder   porous cylinder (for $t \ge 0$)

12.10. Photobleaching, a process that is normally undesirable, can be exploited to determine the diffusion coefficient of a molecule in a particular tissue. A tissue is first made fluorescent by flooding the tissue with the molecule of interest that has been fluorescently labeled. Then, using a laser, a small spherical region is "photo-bleached," meaning that the laser damages the molecules, and they lose all their fluorescence in that region. Fluorescence is slowly regained in that region as other non-denatured fluorescent molecules diffuse into the bleached region.

(a) We wish to examine the diffusion coefficient of fibrinogen in corneal stroma. After saturating the cornea with fluorescently labeled fibrinogen, a small spherical region 30 μm in radius is "photobleached," and then the fluorescence recovery is monitored. It takes approximately 30 s for the center of this region to recover its fluorescence to 50% of its pre-bleached value. What is the diffusion coefficient of the fibrinogen in normal corneal stroma? You may assume that the concentration of fluorescent macromolecules at the edge of the spherical region remains constant at its pre-bleached value during this process.

(b) Now assume another photobleaching process like in part (a), but using a much more powerful laser that not only photobleaches the fluorescent fibrinogen but also destroys the cornea in the 30-μm spherical region and just leaves it as a material that has effectively the same properties as water. At the surface of this spherical region, a denatured collagen membrane that has a very, very low permeability is left. Assume that the flux of fluorescent fibrinogen through this membrane is $j = h_m(C_{cornea} - C_s)$, where C_{cornea} is the pre-bleached concentration of fluorescent fibrinogen in the cornea and C_s is the concentration of fluorescent fibrinogen at the inner surface of the spherical region, just at the surface. Assuming that $h_m = 2 \times 10^{-7}$ cm/s and that the diffusion coefficient of fibrinogen in water is 5×10^{-7} cm²/s, how long will it take for the fluorescence at the center of this region to recover to 50% of its pre-bleached value?

12.11. Drugs are sometimes delivered using a slow-release formulation, e.g. round, porous polymeric particles in which the drug is impregnated. These particles are sometimes made of denatured collagen that is cross-linked using glutaraldehyde. We are interested in the process by which collagen in these particles becomes cross-linked.

Consider a spherical particle of denatured collagen of radius $R = 0.2$ cm. To cross-link this network in place, the particles are placed into glutaraldehyde solution ($c_\infty = 0.04$ g/ml). We are interested in knowing how long the particles must be in this solution in order for the glutaraldehyde to cross-link the collagen.

Assume that the reaction between the glutaraldehyde and the collagen is instantaneous, and that the glutaraldehyde has a diffusion coefficient of 3×10^{-6} cm²/s in these polymer networks. Assume that the reaction is complete when the glutaraldehyde concentration at a location has risen to $c = 0.01$ g/ml.

(a) First consider the case when the process is very slow such that the mass-transfer coefficient characterizing transport from the glutaraldehyde to the surface of the particles is very small ($h_m = 2 \times 10^{-7}$ cm/s), where $j = h_m[C_\infty - C(r = R, t)]$. Determine the minimum time necessary for the reaction to go to completion everywhere inside the particle.

(b) Now let the mixing rate be more rapid such that h_m is greatly increased. What is the least amount of time that will be necessary in order for the reaction to go to completion everywhere inside the particle?

12.12. In a bioreactor, one method of supplying oxygen is to have air-filled bubbles rise up through the culture medium in which cells are suspended, providing oxygen to the cells as the bubbles rise. The medium is a very viscous solution ($\mu = 25$ cP, $\rho = 1.06$ g/cm^3) that helps keep the cells suspended. Assume that the bubbles have a diameter of 1 mm and that this diameter remains constant as a bubble rises at constant velocity. Further assume that the oxygen is taken up so rapidly by the cells that the oxygen concentration in solution and at the surface of the bubble is always negligible, and that the mass transfer coefficient at the surface of the bubble is 0.02 cm/s.

If the bubbles originally contain 20% oxygen, how deep should the tank be so that 75% of the oxygen in each bubble is delivered to the solution by the time the bubble reaches the free surface of the culture medium in the bioreactor? The diffusivity of oxygen in the culture medium is 1.7×10^{-5} cm^2/s, and the diffusivity of oxygen in air (20% oxygen) is 0.1778 cm^2/s. The bioreactor is at a temperature of 37 °C.

12.13. Age-related macular degeneration is a disease of the retina (at the back of the eye). In a proposed new treatment for the disease, a small, transparent, soluble pellet that contains a drug is put in the center of the eye (in the center of the vitreous humor), and the drug diffuses back to the retina. The diffusion coefficient of this drug in the vitreous humor is 1×10^{-7} cm^2/s.

Assume that the eye can be modeled as a sphere with a radius of 1 cm, and that the pellet has a radius of 3 mm. The concentration of drug in the dissolving pellet is

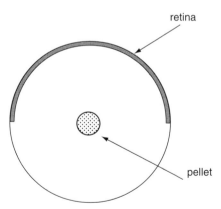

10 mg/ml. You can ignore what happens in the front half of the eye. The thickness of the retina can be neglected.

(a)   Estimate very roughly how long it will be before the drug first reaches the retina.

(b)   Once the drug reaches the retina, any drug that is not taken up by the retina is rapidly removed by the choroid (immediately behind the retina). Essentially there is no drug at the back of the eye ($C = 0$). Assuming that ALL of the drug leaves the eye through the choroid, <u>estimate</u> how long it will take before all of the drug is removed from the eye. You may treat the pellet size as constant and thus treat the problem as quasi-steady-state. You may neglect any mass-transfer resistance due to diffusion of the drug within the pellet.

(c)   How could this drug-delivery strategy be improved?

12.14. The tear film bathes the cornea and protects it from drying out. Every 5 s or so, a blink occurs, replenishing the liquid film to a thickness of 5 μm. Assume that at the end of each blink the air surrounding the tear film is entirely dry.

(a)   Find the fraction of the tear film that evaporates during this period of 5 s. The diffusion coefficient of water in air is 0.26 cm^2/s and the vapor pressure of water at 35 °C, the approximate temperature of the cornea, is such as to create a water-vapor concentration in the air at the surface of the tear film of 4×10^{-5} g/cm^3. (Note that in reality the situation is more complex. There is a thin oil film that "floats" on the surface of the tear film that inhibits evaporation.)

(b)   Compare your answer with that to Problem 4.13, and comment on the comparison.

12.15. ATP is produced by the mitochondria and used by the other organelles within the cell. Transport of ATP to these organelles is passive, i.e. by diffusion, and the purpose of this question is to find out how rapidly that transport can occur. Consider a simple one-dimensional system where $C = C(x, t)$. This is an acceptable model for treating diffusion between a row of mitochondria and a contractile set of actin–myosin fibers, such as is typically found in muscle cells (see the figure overleaf).

Let the average distance between the fibers and the mitochondria be L, and assume that initially the concentration of ATP is uniformly 5 mM everywhere within the cell. At $t = 0$ the muscle contracts, causing the concentration of ATP in the cytoplasm immediately adjacent to the fibers to drop rapidly to zero (or at least approximately to zero) and remain there while the muscle is contracted. The concentration of ATP in the surrounding cytoplasm between the mitochondria and fibers then drops in an unsteady fashion. To a good approximation, you can assume that the mitochondria act to maintain the local ATP concentration at their surface at 5 mM.

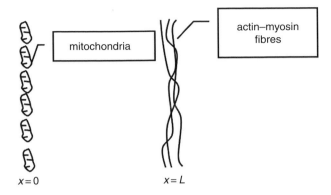

(a) Write down the boundary and initial conditions implied by this scenario, and the differential equation that must be satisfied in the domain $0 < x < L$.

(b) If the fibers are contracted for long enough, the concentration of ATP in the domain $0 < x < L$ will reach a steady-state distribution. If $D = 4.5 \times 10^{-10}$ m^2/s for ATP, and $L = 0.5$ μm, estimate how long the muscle cells would have to be contracted for in order for the concentration of ATP in the cytoplasm around the muscle fiber to have reached a steady-state distribution.

(c) What is the steady-state concentration distribution, $C(x)$, that will be reached?

(d) Sketch graphs of (i) $C(x, t)$ and (ii) $j(t)$, the flux of ATP from the mitochondria. From [2].

12.16. Consider a spherical pellet (original radius a_0) made of a polymer of concentration C_0. This pellet is dissolving in a large fluid bath that originally contains no polymer in solution. Owing to the pellet dissolving, the concentration of polymer in the fluid immediately adjacent to the pellet is $0.1C_0$. Assume that the pellet dissolves very slowly, i.e. that its radius $a(t)$ changes very slowly with time (a quasi-steady process).

(a) After a transient period, the concentration of polymer around the pellet, $C(r)$, $r > a$, reaches a quasi-steady state with the only time-dependence being the slowly changing parameter $a(t)$. Find this distribution for $C_{ss}[r, a(t)]$.

(b) Use this steady-state distribution to help you find the unsteady solution $C(r, t)$, $r > a$, by assuming that $C(r, t) = C_{ss}[r, a(t)] f(\eta)$, where $\eta = (r - a(t))/(2\sqrt{Dt})$, while continuing to treat $a(t)$ as a constant.

(c) Using this solution, find the rate (J, mass/time) at which the pellet is dissolving and estimate the time at which the quasi-steady solution would give a good approximation of this rate.

12.17. Consider an experiment in which vascular endothelial growth factor (VEGF) is delivered to the basal side of a monolayer of endothelial cells through a gel layer

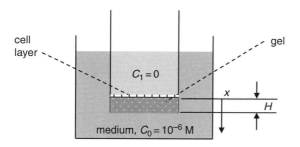

of thickness H. The concentration of VEGF above the cells (C_1) is zero, and the concentration is C_0 below the gel. The cells in the surface layer are connected to one another by very tight junctions, and you can assume that there is no diffusion through this narrow layer. The gel initially contains no VEGF.

You may assume that (i) the lower fluid volume is initially well mixed and sufficiently large that the concentration (C_0) far from the cells does not change during the time-course of the experiment, (ii) there is no internal binding of VEGF to the gel, (iii) the equilibrium partition coefficient K between the gel and the medium is 0.8 (defined here as the concentration of protein in the gel divided by the concentration in solution, across an interface at equilibrium), and (iv) the uptake of VEGF by the cells is so small that it can be neglected.

(a) Determine how long it will be before the cells are exposed to a VEGF concentration of $0.05C_0$. Call this time $t_{0.05}$.
(b) Estimate the total amount of VEGF in the gel at time $t_{0.05}$.
(c) Determine an expression for the flux of VEGF entering the bottom of the gel (at $x = H$) that is valid for very short times $t \ll t_{0.05}$.
(d) Using your result from part (c), estimate how much VEGF will enter the gel during the interval $0 \leq t \leq t_{0.05}$.
(e) Compare your answers for parts (b) and (d).

Use the following parameter values:

- $H = 2$ mm
- $C_0 = 10^{-6}$ M
- $D = 10^{-7}$ cm^2/s (diffusivity of VEGF in gel)
- $A = 5$ cm^2 (cross-sectional area of gel perpendicular to the x-direction)

12.18. Aerosols can enter the lung and adsorb onto its surface, potentially leading to a negative impact on health. Consider an individual alveolus (the terminal spherical hollow cavities at the end of the respiratory system) that has a time-averaged radius of 150 μm. The radius of the alveolus decreases from 152.5 to 147.5 μm during normal expiration, and then increases to 152.5 μm during inspiration.

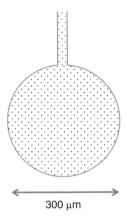

300 µm

During one cycle of inspiration (air entering the lung), assume that one alveolus becomes full of very fine spherical aerosol particles at concentration $C_0 = 1\%$ (by volume). The particles have a diameter of 10 nm and a density of 1 g/ml. You may assume that the alveolus is oriented as shown in the figure, with gravity pointing down.

Assuming that any aerosol particle that hits the alveolar wall will be irreversibly adsorbed, calculate the concentration of particles remaining at the center of the alveolus after an expiration that takes 1.5 s.

12.19. Nerve growth factor (NGF) has been found to be therapeutic in regions of the brain where nerve damage has occurred. One proposed therapy is to place a small round pellet (of initial radius $a_0 = 0.1$ cm) such that NGF is slowly released to the surrounding tissue. We wish to find the region of action of this agent, and how long the pellet will continue to deliver drug to the tissue.

The initial concentration of NGF in the pellet is 1 mg/ml. The diffusion coefficient of the NGF within the pellet ($D_p = 1 \times 10^{-5}$ cm^2/s) is much larger than that in the brain tissue ($D = 1 \times 10^{-7}$ cm^2/s). Thus you may assume that the concentration of NGF remains uniform (but not constant) within the pellet: that is $C(r < a_0, t) = C_p(t)$ and $C_p(t = 0) = C_0 = 1$ mg/ml.

(a) Assume that the brain cells in the tissue where the pellet is to be placed are uniformly distributed and take up the NGF at a rate per unit tissue volume of $\beta C(r, t)$, where $\beta = 10^{-6}$ s^{-1} and $C(r, t)$ is the concentration of NGF at a radius r from the center of the pellet. Find a differential equation that describes $C(r, t)$.

(b) Assume that the differential equation has a solution of the form $C(r, t) = f(t)/r$. Find $f(t)$ for the region $r > a$. Your solution should satisfy appropriate boundary conditions, including the initial condition at $C(r = a_0, t = 0)$. However, your solution will not satisfy the initial condition that $C(r > a_0, t = 0) = 0$.

(c) Now assume that the pellet is actually dissolving such that the radius of the pellet is a function of time, $a(t)$. Assuming your solution for part (b) is still valid, *roughly* estimate how long drug will continue to be delivered to the tissue. Note that β is very small, and therefore the pellet concentration can be assumed to be roughly constant during this process.

(d) In part (c), it was assumed that β was sufficiently small that C_p could be treated as a constant. Using results from above, give a criterion on β for the conditions under which this assumption is reasonable, and evaluate whether these conditions are satisfied for this problem.

12.20. Treatment of AIDS requires careful monitoring of the viral load in the blood, which can be done by measuring the level of the HIV protein p24 in the blood. This measurement involves a step in which the p24 binds to the surface of nanospheres (radius $a = 40$ nm) that are coated with an antibody to the p24. The antibody is denoted a-p24, and the concentration of unbound a-p24 on the surface of the nanospheres is denoted Γ_a. We are interested in the rate at which the p24 binds to the nanospheres.

Consider one such nanosphere in a solution of p24 at a concentration C_0. At the surface of the microsphere, the p24 reacts with the antibody according to the following first-order reaction:

$$p24 + a\text{-}p24 \leftrightarrow p24/a\text{-}p24$$

with the forward rate being proportional to the concentration of p24 at the surface of the nanosphere, $C_p(r = a, t)$, and the concentration of a-p24 on the nanosphere, $\Gamma_a(t)$. The forward rate constant is k_1. The backward reaction rate is proportional to the concentration of the p24/a-p24 complex on the surface of the nanoparticles, $\Gamma_{p/a}$, and has a rate constant of k_2.

(a) Write an expression for the net rate of formation of p24/a-p24 ($d\Gamma_{p/a}/dt$) as a function of $C_p(r = a, t)$ and $\Gamma_a(t)$. Give the dimensions of each of the terms.

(b) Give a criterion for whether this process is limited by the forward reaction rate (k_1) or by diffusion.

(c) Now assume that the process is diffusion-limited and thus, for short time, further assume that the concentration of p24 at the surface of the nanosphere drops to nearly zero as it is adsorbed by the nanoparticle. If the diffusion coefficient of the p24 is D, find the rate of mass transfer to the surface of the nanosphere at this time.

(d) For these conditions, find an expression for $d\Gamma_{p/a}/dt$ in terms of C_0, D, k_1, and k_2.

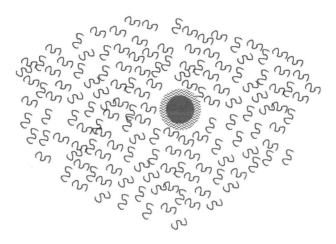

12.21. Sodium fluorescein (NaF) diffuses through sclera with a steady-state diffusion coefficient of 1.3×10^{-6} cm^2/s. However, NaF can also bind to the scleral tissue (presumably to the collagen fibrils), and this can transiently slow down the effective diffusion (until the binding surfaces are saturated). This binding process can be characterized by the following equilibrium relationship:

$$C_b = \frac{B_{max} C_f}{K_D + C_f}$$

where the concentration of bound NaF is C_b, the concentration of free fluorescein is C_f, the maximum binding capacity of the tissue at any location is $B_{max} = 80$ mM, and the equilibrium dissociation constant is $K_D = 2.5$ mM [12]. The binding of NaF to the tissue can be assumed to be instantaneous.

(a) Considering unsteady diffusion, find an expression for the effective diffusion coefficient at any location as a function of C_f at that location. (Hint: let C_T be the total concentration of NaF at any location (bound and free); find an expression for $\partial C_T / \partial t$ at any location.)

(b) Let a NaF depot of concentration 10 mM be placed onto the surface of the sclera. Assume the depot is large enough that its concentration does not change with time. Roughly estimate how long it will take before a detectable amount of fluorescein crosses the sclera if the thickness of the sclera is 0.5 mm. (Since D_{eff} depends on C_f, you should consider what diffusion coefficient will best characterize this process.) Compare this duration with how long it would take if the NaF did not bind to the sclera.

12.22. The study of heat transfer in the human body is complicated by the circulation. While equations have been developed to model the physiological heat-transfer process (e.g. the bioheat equation), a simpler approach is to determine an "effective thermal conductivity" that very roughly accounts for how the circulation increases the rate of heat transfer through tissue.

Consider a model of the radial temperature distribution in the torso of a resting person. Model the torso as a cylinder 0.5 m long with a radius of 15 cm. Let the rate of metabolic heat generation in the body be 1200 W/m^3. Let the density of the body be $\rho = 1000$ kg/m^3, and let the heat capacity be $c = 3500$ J/kg per °C.

(a)   If the steady-state core temperature is 37 °C and the skin temperature is 34.5 °C, calculate the effective thermal conductivity (k_{eff}) of the torso. Compare the calculated value with the thermal conductivity of water to determine the extent to which the circulation has increased the thermal conductivity of the tissue.

(b)   Define the heat-transfer coefficient as $h = Q/[A(T_{\text{skin}} - T_{\text{air}})]$, where Q is the heat flux from the torso to the air and A is the surface area of the torso. Letting the room temperature be 21 °C, find h for steady-state conditions, and also find the Biot number, using the torso radius.

(c)   Whole-body cooling is sometimes done before heart surgery in order to slow down cellular metabolic processes, thus reducing tissue demand for oxygen and permitting longer surgical times. To cool the person sufficiently quickly, a heart–lung machine is used in which the blood is directly cooled. After the surgical procedure, rewarming is sometimes done passively.

Consider a person cooled before surgery to 34 °C, and then after surgery, put into a room at 23 °C to rewarm passively. Let h and k_{eff} be the same as their baseline values. Assume that, because of thermal regulation (which is inhibited during surgery), the rate of metabolic heat generation in the body is 1500 W/m^3 and remains at this elevated value until the body temperature has returned to 37 °C, at which time the internal heat generation will drop.

Assuming a low Biot number (a coarse assumption), estimate how long it would take for the core temperature of the body to warm from 34 °C to 37 °C. Comparing the actual Biot number computed from part (b) with the assumption of a low Biot number, will the heating time that you computed be an over-estimate or an under-estimate?

12.23. On cold winter days, it is necessary to heat up the car before driving, especially to warm up the windshield glass so that it does not fog up and obscure vision. Consider a very cold day such that the windshield glass (of thermal conductivity $k = 1$ W/m per °C, density $\rho = 2500$ kg/m^3, and heat capacity $c = 840$ J/kg per °C) is at a temperature of 10 °F. The windshield is 0.5 cm thick. (Note that 1 W = 1 J/s.)

When turning on the defroster, let the temperature of the air blowing onto the inside of the windshield be 90 °F, and let the heat-transfer coefficient of this air to the windshield be 50 W/m^2 per °C everywhere on the windshield (this is not a good assumption, but it greatly simplifies the problem). Since the car is not moving and the air outside the car is stationary, you may assume that on its outside surface, the window is essentially insulated.

(a) Determine how long it will take until the temperature of the window is everywhere greater than 32 °F.

(b) Now consider that a new "super glass" (made of industrial diamonds) that has a very high thermal conductivity ($k = 1200$ W/m per °C), with its other properties the same as regular glass, has been developed. Determine how long it will take until the temperature of the window is everywhere greater than 32 °F.

12.24. Consider a paper cup (with negligible heat capacity and a thermal conductivity of 0.05 W/m per K) whose walls are 0.5 mm thick. Let the coffee inside be at a temperature of 80° C. If the threshold temperature for pain is when the skin temperature has risen to 45 °C, estimate how long you can hold the coffee cup until it becomes painful. Let the skin have a thermal diffusivity of $\alpha = 1.6 \times 10^{-7}$ m^2/s and a thermal conductivity of 0.2 W/m per K. You may neglect the effects of the circulation in the skin.

13 Convection of mass and heat

(20 mass-convection problems; 1 heat-convection problem)

13.1. A fluorescently labeled molecule (with a diffusion coefficient of $1 \times 10^{-6}\,\mathrm{cm^2/s}$) is released into the upstream end of a small blood vessel of diameter 100 μm and length 2 mm. The flow rate of blood passing through this vessel is 0.3 μl/min. Roughly estimate how long it should take before the molecule can be detected at the downstream end of the blood vessel.

13.2. Transport of nutrients, growth factors, and other molecules to tissues frequently takes place through the capillary wall. In many capillaries, there are tiny gaps between endothelial cells that allow both diffusion and convection of solutes across the vessel wall. Consider a particular endothelium in which the gaps between the cells are characterized by the following dimensions: $L = 1$ μm long, $h = 200$ nm high, and $W = 10$ nm in width (the last dimension is the distance between the two cells; see the figure below). The fluid in this gap is at 37 °C, and has the same properties as physiologic saline.

Let the average pressure in the capillary be 45 mm Hg, and let the pressure in the tissue be 0 mm Hg (ignore osmotic effects). Consider a small solute that has a

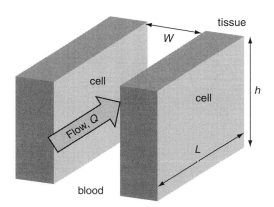

diffusion coefficient of 1×10^{-5} cm^2/s. Does this solute pass across the endothelium by diffusion, or is it primarily carried by the flow?

13.3. It is well known that coughing and sneezing can transmit germs and viruses. It has been proposed that whistling can do this too. We explore this possibility here.

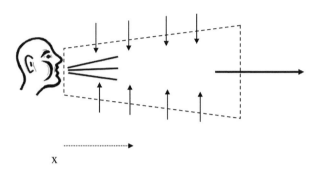

x

Consider a person whistling. Let the flow rate of air out of the mouth and into the atmosphere be Q_0 and assume steady flow. Let the air density be ρ, and treat the fluid flow as inviscid. The air leaving the mouth is a cylindrical jet that expands with a small angle α such that the radius of the jet is $R(x) = R_0 + \alpha x$, where x is the distance from the mouth. As this turbulent jet flows outward, it "entrains" air in the direction of flow. You may assume the air to be incompressible.

(a) Find the flow rate in the jet as a function of x and the other given quantities. (Note that, owing to the entrainment of air, the flow rate in the jet increases with x; what fluid-mechanical quantity is conserved in this flow?)

(b) Now consider that the air exiting from the mouth contains virus particles. Let the concentration of these virus particles in this exiting jet be b particles per unit volume. Find the concentration of virus particles in the jet as a function of distance from the mouth. Assume that the air surrounding the jet is virus-particle-free and neglect the effect of the virus particles on the air flow.

13.4. Consider a solution containing a small solute and larger particulates. The solution is to be passed through a filter to remove the particulates while the small solute passes freely through the filter. Denote this solute by "A," and assume that it is present in the feed solution at a low concentration $C_{A,0}$ and has diffusion coefficient D_A. The fluid passing through the filter mixes quickly with a flowing stream on the downstream side of the filter in which the concentration of A is zero.

(a) If the filter pores are cylindrical with radius R and length L, and a constant pressure drop of Δp is maintained across the filter, derive a criterion solely in terms of given quantities, in order to determine whether the transport of solute A across the filter is dominated by convection or diffusion.

(b) A solution of glucose (of concentration 1 mg/ml with a diffusion coefficient of 6×10^{-5} cm^2/s) in physiologic saline at 20 °C is being filtered to remove bacteria. The filter has a total area of 4 cm^2, a pore diameter of 0.4 μm, a thickness of 10 μm, and a porosity of 5%. The pressure drop driving flow through the filter is 100 mm Hg. Find the rate of transport of glucose through the filter into this stream. You may ignore any effects of the bacteria plugging up the filter.

13.5. Nutrients and fluid can pass out of blood vessels and into the surrounding tissue by passing through narrow spaces between endothelial cells. We are interested in determining the steady-state flux of glucose through these junctions in the venous end of a capillary bed. Consider an endothelial cell of thickness 1.5 μm. Let one of the junctions between this cell and the next be 10 nm in thickness. Let the distance between such junctions be 100 nm, such that fluid and nutrients can pass through a slit channel that is 10 nm high, 100 nm wide, and 1.5 μm long (see the figure below). The fluid within this channel has the properties of physiologic saline at 37 °C.

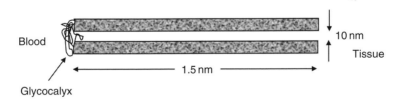

The entrance to this channel is covered with the glycocalyx of the cell, which allows glucose to freely enter this channel, but prevents the proteins in the blood from entering. The osmotic pressure of the proteins (primarily albumin) in the blood in this venular capillary is 20 mm Hg and the hydrostatic pressure in this venular capillary is 5 mm Hg (the osmotic pressure and hydrostatic pressure in the surrounding tissue can both be assumed to be negligible). The concentration of glucose in the blood is 1 mg/ml, while the concentration of glucose in the tissue is zero. The diffusion coefficient of glucose in the slit channel is 5×10^{-6} cm^2/s. The uptake of glucose by the cells can be neglected.

Estimate the flux of glucose passing through one of these slit channels from the blood to the tissue. Clearly state and justify all assumptions that you make.

13.6. Consider the steady diffusion of a ligand within the lateral intercellular space (LIS) between two cells. You may assume that the ligand concentration $C(x)$ depends only upon x, and that the diffusion coefficient for this ligand is D. The dimensions of the LIS are its widths, w_1 and w_2, and height $H_1 + H_2$ as shown in the sketch below. You may assume that there is no exchange normal to the sketch, so that all the transport is one-dimensional. You may also assume that the height H_1 is negligible compared with H_2, and thus the cleft is essentially the width w_2 for its entire length. However, the small opening at the top (width w_1) is sufficiently small that the ligand can neither enter the LIS nor leave at the top.

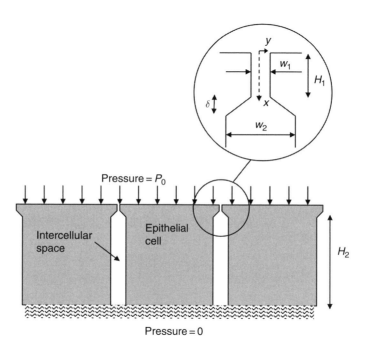

The ligand enters the LIS as a result of the ligand being shed from the cell membrane into the LIS, which is assumed to occur at a constant rate R from the two cell membranes (R is in moles per unit membrane area per unit time). Give all answers in terms of given quantities.

(a) Assume that there is no flow through the LIS. Find the concentration distribution of ligand in the LIS, and find the rate (per unit depth) at which ligand leaves the bottom of the LIS ($x = H_1 + H_2 \approx H_2$). You may assume (for this part only) that the ligand is rapidly removed when it leaves the LIS at $x = H_1 + H_2$ and thus $C(x = H_1 + H_2 \approx H_2) = 0$.

(b) Now let the cell walls also secrete fluid into the LIS at a rate q (volume/time per membrane area). There is also a small flow (Q_0, volume/time per unit depth) entering the LIS at $x = 0$ flowing in the positive x-direction. Find the concentration distribution of ligand in the LIS, and find the rate (per unit depth) at which ligand leaves the bottom of the LIS ($x = H_1 + H_2 \approx H_2$).

You may assume that the convective flow in the LIS (in the x-direction) is much greater than diffusional transport. Also give the conditions necessary for this assumption to hold. (Hint: it will be helpful to derive the one-dimensional convection–diffusion equation; directly using the two-dimensional convection–diffusion equation is a little harder than it looks at first.)

13.7. Drug delivery through the skin can be done by placing a drug-saturated patch on the skin. Consider such a patch 5 cm × 5 cm × 2 mm. We wish to consider the diffusion of this drug across the dermis and then into a dense bed of capillaries underlying this tissue.

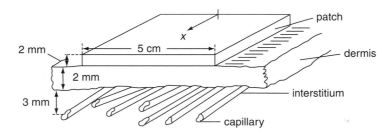

One benefit of saturating the patch with drug is that the concentration of drug at its surface remains nearly constant at $C_p = 5$ mg/ml until the drug is used up. The rate of blood flow through the capillary bed is 5×10^{-4} ml/min. The drug's diffusivity across the dermis is 5×10^{-8} cm²/s, while that in the interstitium surrounding the capillaries is 8×10^{-6} cm²/s. The capillaries are oriented primarily as shown in the figure (which is not drawn to scale), and the drug can freely penetrate the capillary walls. The dermis is 2 mm in thickness.

(a)   Derive an expression for the concentration of drug in a capillary as a function of x, the distance from the beginning of the patch in the direction in which the blood in the capillaries is flowing. You may assume that the concentration of drug in the capillaries is a function only of x and does not vary with radial position within the capillary.

(b)   Estimate how long the patch will last if it is initially loaded with 50 mg of drug.

13.8. As a controlled-release drug-delivery system, a small, porous sphere is surgically implanted into the body, and connected via a catheter to a syringe. Drug is delivered to the sphere in solution at a constant volume flow rate of $Q\,\mathrm{m^3/s}$. The concentration of drug in the delivered solution is C_D. Drug-containing solution exits through the porous surface at radius R, uniformly over the entire surface area. You may assume that the diffusion coefficient for the drug in the organ tissue is D_D, and that the tissue is completely isotropic and homogeneous.

(a) Find an expression for the flow velocity of solvent, v_r, as a function of the radial distance r from the center of the sphere, for $r > R$.

(b) Neglecting the convective flow, just for now, and assuming that the drug concentration at the surface of the sphere $(r = R)$ is C_D and constant, find an expression for the steady-state concentration distribution of the drug, making an appropriate assumption regarding the concentration of drug at large distances from the point of delivery.

(c) Find an expression for the ratio between the rate of transport of drug by convection, and the rate of transport by diffusion, as a function of the radial distance r, for $r > R$. This represents the Péclet number for this situation. Explain what this tells you about the relative importance of convection and diffusion close to the sphere as compared with far from it.

(d) Solve for $C(r)$ for $r > R$ and compare your answer with the results of part (b)

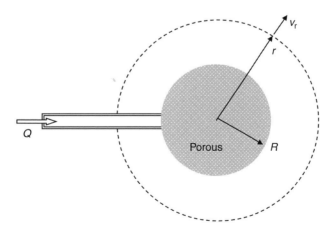

13.9. A protein solution is being concentrated by filtration. You may assume that the solution consists of a single protein in water, that the membrane freely passes the water, and that the membrane prevents most of the protein from passing through. Specifically, the amount of protein retained by the filter is quantified by the filter rejection coefficient, R, which is defined by

$$1 - R = \frac{\text{protein mass flux passing through filter}}{v\,C_0}$$

where v is the magnitude of the mass-average velocity. $C(x)$ is the protein mass concentration, and C_0 is the value of C at $x = 0$, i.e. at the filter surface. Note that, as R approaches 1, less and less protein passes through the filter. The solution can be assumed to be dilute everywhere.

(a) Draw a suitable control volume and show by a mass balance that, at steady state, the protein mass flux leaking through the membrane must equal the product vC_∞, where C_∞ is the protein density in the feed solution far from the membrane.

(b) Using the same control volume and the definition of R, show that $C_0 = C_\infty/(1 - R)$.

(c) If the protein's diffusion coefficient in water is $D = 6 \times 10^{-6}$ cm^2/s, $C_\infty = 10$ μg/ml, and $R = 98\%$, determine the steady-state protein mass concentration, $C(x)$, at $x = 0.001$ cm. The solution is pumped at a steady flow rate of $Q = 0.1$ ml/s through a membrane with surface area 5 cm^2. This part of the question requires you to compute $C(x)$.

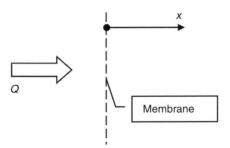

13.10. A microbial system is used to produce a protein, A, which is useful as a pharmaceutical. Unfortunately, the microbe also produces a second protein, B, which is toxic. The protein B is similar in size to the protein A, and thus it is difficult to filter out.

One method by which to remove protein B is to perfuse the solution containing both proteins through a gel in which is immobilized an enzyme that breaks down protein B at a rate (per unit volume) of $\dot{\varepsilon} = -K C_B(x)$, where $C_B(x)$ is the concentration of protein B at a location x (see the figure overleaf). Let the gel have a thickness L, and assume the fluid flow velocity through the gel to be uniform and equal to V. Let the diffusion coefficient of protein B in the gel be D_B. Let $C_B(x = 0) = C_0$, where $x = 0$ is the beginning of the gel. Note that the gel is stationary and not transported by the flow.

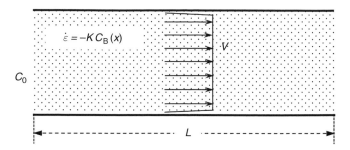

(a)   Assume the gel is sufficiently thick that L is effectively infinite. Find $C_B(x)$.

(b)   Find a dimensionless parameter that characterizes whether diffusion or convection is dominant in this problem (again assuming that L is effectively infinite).

(c)   Find $C_B(x)$ for the case when convection is dominant and diffusion does not play a role in the problem.

(d)   Let $V = 0.1$ mm/s, $D_B = 1 \times 10^{-7}$ cm^2/s and $K = 0.1$ s^{-1}. How long should L be in order for the concentration of protein B to be reduced 100-fold when the fluid emerges from the gel at $x = L$?

13.11. Consider a filter of area A that rejects a macromolecule. A mass M of the macromolecule with diffusion coefficient D is injected upstream of the filter in saline. The macromolecule has a diffusion coefficient in saline that varies with its concentration, C, such that $D(C) = D_0 + D_1C$.

(a)   If the saline flows through the filter at a flow rate of Q, find a differential equation that describes the steady-state distribution $C(x)$ of the macromolecules upstream of the filter where $-\infty < x \leq 0$, and find the boundary conditions or constraints that this equation must satisfy. You may assume that in the region where $C(x)$ is significantly different from zero, the velocity is everywhere equal to Q/A (because of the presence of the filter).

(b)   Find $C_0 = C(x = 0)$ in two limits: (i) $D_0 \gg D_1C_0$ and (ii) $D_0 \ll D_1C_0$. (Hint: you do not need to find $C(x)$.)

13.12. In a confined-compression experiment, as is often performed on a sample of tissue such as cartilage to determine its properties, a cylindrical sample is placed inside of a container (of height $H(t)$ and radius R, $H \ll R$) and compressed from above by a tight-fitting piston (see the figure on the next page). Assuming that the piston and the bottom of the container are non-porous (no flow or transport occurs) but that the lateral, cylindrical walls are porous, answer the following questions to analyze the transport of protein during an experiment in which the sample is being transiently compressed at a constant rate of $U = -dH/dt$. You may leave your answers in terms of U and the instantaneous value of $H(t)$.

(a) First consider only diffusion, and let a protein be produced uniformly within the tissue at a rate S (per unit volume). Obtain an expression for the concentration of protein, $C(r)$, as a function of r (the radial distance from the center). Let the diffusion coefficient of the protein be D and let the concentration of protein at the porous side walls ($r = R$) be C_{wall}. Assume quasi-steady conditions.

(b) Find an expression for the radial velocity $v_r(r, t)$ of the fluid in the chamber under the assumption that the flow is purely radial ($v_\theta = v_z = 0$).

(c) Now, assume again that the protein is being produced uniformly within the tissue at a rate of S (per unit volume), but now neglect diffusion and consider only convection.

    (i) Show that there is no steady (or quasi-steady) solution that solves the convection–diffusion equation and conclude that $C = f(r, t)$.

    (ii) Let $C(r, t) = T(t) + g(r)$. Letting $C(r, t = 0) = C_0$, find $C(r, t)$.

(d) Consider now a situation in which the initial concentration of C is not spatially uniform, so the solution from part (c) does not hold. Let the radius of the container be $R = 5$ cm, $H = 0.5$ cm, $D = 10^{-10}$ m²/s, $S = 10^{-6}$ mol/m³ per s, and $dH/dt = -10^{-7}$ m/s. Determine whether the concentration distribution in the chamber will be dominated by convective or diffusive effects.

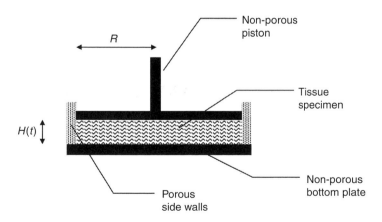

13.13. A cylindrical bioreactor consists of cells embedded in an extracellular matrix. These cells produce significant quantities of a small soluble peptide that is of therapeutic use, but also produce a large soluble protein that is not of utility. We wish to collect the peptide, while leaving the large protein behind. This protein has a diffusion coefficient in the extracellular matrix of $D = 6 \times 10^{-7}$ cm^2/s and a molecular weight of 45 kD.

The bioreactor has culture medium (with oxygen and nutrients) entering at its center (at $r = R_1 = 0.5$ cm) and leaving at the periphery ($r = R_2 = 2$ cm); the height of this narrow cylindrical chamber is $h = 0.2$ cm. A filter present at the periphery allows the small peptide to pass through freely (together with the culture medium), but prevents the large protein from passing through the filter. The flow through the reactor is driven by a pressure difference of 100 mm Hg. This generates an initial flow rate of culture medium through the bioreactor of $Q_0 = 0.050$ ml/min. For parts (a)–(d) you may assume that this flow rate is constant. The cells are uniformly embedded in the extracellular matrix, and produce the large protein at a rate of $\alpha = 3 \times 10^{-4}$ mg/s per cm^3 (this is per reactor volume, not per cell volume). The culture medium has the same properties as physiologic saline.

(a) Derive a differential equation that describes the distribution of the large protein in the bioreactor, $C(r, t)$, as a function of the radius r, time t, Q, and D.

(b) Because the diffusion coefficient of the large protein is so low, this protein accumulates at the outer periphery. Except in this narrow region near the filter (of thickness δ), the bioreactor reaches a steady-state concentration profile, $C(r)$, for the large protein. Neglecting diffusion, and neglecting the rejection of this protein at the filter, find $C(r)$ for $R_1 < r < (R_2 - \delta)$.

(c) Give a criterion for neglecting diffusion in part (b) and determine whether the criterion is satisfied for this problem.

(d) Near the rejecting filter, diffusion of the large protein cannot be neglected. Estimate the thickness of this region.

(e) While the flow rate remains relatively constant at Q_0 for quite some time, eventually the flow rate begins to drop. What causes the flow rate to drop?

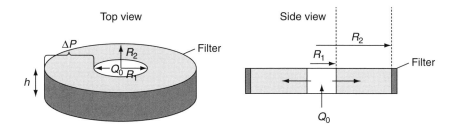

13.14. A solution of bacteria is placed into a cylindrical chamber (see the diagram) at a temperature of 25 °C. A very slow flow of culture medium (originating at the center of the chamber) provides oxygen and nutrients to the cells. The culture medium has the same flow properties as physiologic saline. At the outer radius of this chamber ($r = R_0$) is a filter with a sufficiently small pore size to prevent the cells from leaving the chamber, but which allows the medium to pass. We are interested in determining the flow rate of medium in order to adequately provide for the needs of the cells, but do not want the flow rate to be so high that the cells all pile up on the filter.

The bacterial cells are round and have a diameter of 0.4 μm. You may assume them to have the same density as the medium. The radius of the cylindrical chamber is 3 mm and the height of the fluid layer is 1 mm. The radius of the inlet to the flow chamber (R_I) is 0.3 mm.

(a) What physical phenomenon allows the cells to stay in solution away from the filter?

(b) <u>Estimate</u> the maximum flow rate of buffer for which the cells do not all pile up on the filter.

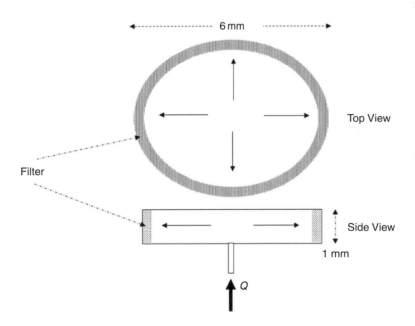

13.15. Consider a tissue bioreactor consisting of hepatocytes embedded in an extracellular matrix placed into a long cylindrical tube of radius R and length L. Oxygen and nutrients, and other moieties, are brought to the cells by an axial flow that passes through this artificial tissue at a flow rate of Q. Owing to the presence of the extracellular matrix, the velocity V is uniform everywhere in the tube (except immediately adjacent to the tube wall due to the no-slip boundary condition, but that can be ignored for this problem).

The cells are embedded in the matrix at a concentration of n cells per unit volume and each cell takes up glucose at a rate of $sC(x)$ mol/s, where $C(x)$ is the concentration of glucose in the tube at a location x. The fluid entering the tube has a glucose concentration of C_0. The diffusion coefficient of glucose in the matrix is D. We would like to find the maximum length of the tube such that all cells are exposed to a glucose concentration $\geq 0.05 C_0$.

(a) Using a differential control volume extending from x to $x + dx$, derive a differential equation for $C(x)$.

(b) Use the species-transport equation to derive this equation.

(c) Consider the limit when the flow rate Q is high enough that the diffusional terms can be neglected. Solve for the concentration distribution, $C(x)$.

(d) Determine the maximum length of the tube (L_{max}) such that all of the cells are exposed to a glucose concentration of at least $0.05 C_0$.

(e) Now consider the limit when Q is sufficiently small that glucose transport to the cells is dominated by diffusion. Solve for the concentration distribution, $C(x)$, assuming that $C(x = \infty)$ is zero. Find what the maximum value of x is such that $C(x) > 0.05 C_0$.

(f) Give a criterion (in terms of known quantities) for when you can neglect diffusion.

13.16. A suspension of cells, extracellular matrix, and saline is placed between two circular disks (each of radius 1.5 cm) that are spaced a distance $\delta = 0.1$ cm apart. Oxygen is consumed by this cell–matrix mixture at a rate per unit volume given by $S = 7 \times 10^{-9}$ g/ml per s. Oxygen diffuses through this cell–matrix mixture with $D = 2 \times 10^{-5}$ cm^2/s. Assume steady-state conditions.

(a) Let this cell–matrix mixture occupy the region $r < b$ between the plates for $b = 0.5$ cm (see the figure below). If the oxygen concentration at the outer edge of the cell–matrix mixture is maintained at $C_0 = 8.4 \times 10^{-6}$ g/ml, determine whether an adequate amount of oxygen will be supplied to all cells and, if not, at which locations cell death would be expected.

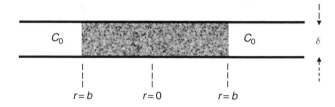

(b) To ensure that an adequate amount of oxygen is supplied to all cells, a very slow flow of saline ($Q = 3.8$ μl/min) is supplied at $r = b$ and is removed at $r = a$

(see the figure below), where $a = 0.1$ cm. The cell–matrix mixture fills the region $a < r < b$. The saline entering the cell–matrix mixture has an oxygen concentration of C_0. Determine whether there will be an adequate supply of oxygen to all cells and, if not, at which locations cell death is to be expected. You may ignore the influence of diffusion in your calculation, and may assume that the cell–matrix mixture is sufficiently rigid that it is not displaced by the flow.

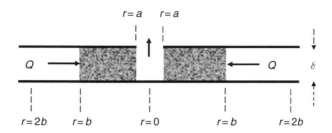

(c) Evaluate whether or not it is reasonable to ignore diffusion in part (b) in determining $C(r)$.

13.17. Consider the Krogh tissue-cylinder model of Problem 11.10. In that problem, the maximum oxygenated radius of a tissue cylinder surrounding a capillary (with anoxia occurring at the outer surface of the cylinder) was determined. The solution depended on the given concentration of oxygen in the capillary. In practice the concentration drops from the arteriolar to the venous end of the capillary. Here, the analysis is revised to take this into account.

Consider a tissue cylinder of radius $R = 20$ μm and of length L surrounding a capillary of radius $a = 5$ μm. Let the flow rate of blood passing through this capillary be 0.02 μl/min, and let it have an oxygen tension entering the capillary of 100 mm Hg (the partial pressure which is equivalent to the concentration of oxygen in the tissue). This tissue uses oxygen at a rate of 180 mm Hg/s (this is a consumption rate per unit volume; check your units), and oxygen diffuses through the tissue with $D = 1.7 \times 10^{-5}$ cm²/s.

You may assume that oxygen in the tissue diffuses only radially, i.e. oxygen diffusion in the axial direction can be neglected, and that the oxygen diffusion coefficient across the endothelial cell layer lining the capillary is comparable to that in the surrounding tissue. The difference between the (greater) oxygen-consumption rate of the endothelial cell layer and that of the surrounding tissue can be neglected.

(a) Using the principle of oxygen conservation, find the flux of oxygen passing from the capillary to the tissue cylinder at any axial location x.

(b) Neglecting entrance effects and axial diffusion, find the average concentration of oxygen in the capillary as a function of x, the distance from the entrance to the capillary.

(c) Now, in the Krogh cylinder model, all tissue within the tissue cylinder is required to have oxygen (there are no anoxic regions). Assuming that the radial concentration gradient is negligible within the capillary (this introduces a small error into the calculation), find how long (L) the tissue cylinder can be for this condition to be satisfied. This location ($r = R$, $x = L$) is known as the "lethal corner."

13.18. A long capillary tube (of radius 1 mm and length 2 m, initially filled with only physiologic saline) is connected to an experiment in which we want to deliver a drug and then determine how quickly the cells can respond to this drug. However, when the drug is introduced at one end of the tube, we know that there will be a delay before the drug reaches the other end of the tube.

To evaluate this delay, we set up an experiment in which the effluent from the capillary tube is delivered to a beaker with a stir bar inside so that the solution is well mixed. We use a spectrophotometer to monitor the concentration of drug inside the beaker. Assume that, at $t = 0$, drug enters the capillary tube at a uniform concentration of C_0 with a flow rate of 1 ml/min. Diffusion can be neglected.

(a) When will the drug first arrive at the end of the tube?

(b) Find the rate at which the drug leaves the tube as a function of time.

(c) Assuming that the beaker is initially empty, predict the concentration of drug in the beaker as a function of time.

(d) If the diffusion coefficient of the drug is 1×10^{-6} cm^2/s, evaluate whether the assumption that one can neglect diffusion is reasonable.

13.19. In a bioreactor system, cells in solution are being transported under steady-state conditions from one reactor tank to another reactor tank through a long rectangular channel. This channel has a height of h, a width W, and a length L ($h \ll W$, $h \ll L$). There are N cells per unit volume, and the cells are distributed uniformly in the solution.

The flow rate of fluid (culture medium and cells) passing through the rectangular channel is Q. Each cell gives off CO_2 at a rate of r (mol/s). CO_2 has a diffusion coefficient of D (cm^2/s). Let $C(x, y)$ be the concentration of CO_2 at any location x, y and let $C_A(x)$ be the flow-averaged concentration of CO_2 at a location x, defined as the flow-wise distance from the channel entry. The Péclet number for CO_2 transport is high.

(a) Calculate the rate (dC_A/dx) at which the average CO_2 concentration would increase in the channel, assuming that the walls of the channel do not adsorb the CO_2.

(b) Now assume that the walls of this channel (at $y = \pm h/2$) adsorb the CO_2 uniformly at a rate of s (mol/s per cm^2). Find what s would have to be in order that the CO_2 concentration not increase $(dC_A/dx = 0)$.

(c) Considering again this case with the walls adsorbing CO_2 such that $dC_A/dx = 0$, the concentration of CO_2 in the center of the tube $(y = 0)$ will be higher than that at the wall $(y = \pm h/2)$. If $C(x, y = 0)$ is given as C_0, find how much greater the CO_2 concentration in the center of the tube is than that at the walls: in other words, find $C(x, y = 0) - C(x, y = h/2)$.

(d) Find the total rate of CO_2 leaving the channel at the exit. (You will need to know the velocity distribution $V_x(y)$, which can be assumed to be fully developed.)

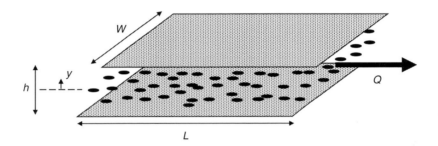

13.20. Characteristic times for biological transport processes are frequently described in terms of a mean residence or transit time. The mean transit time is the average time taken for a substance to pass through a system. If $C(t)$ is the mean concentration of the tracer at the system exit, then the mean transit time is defined as

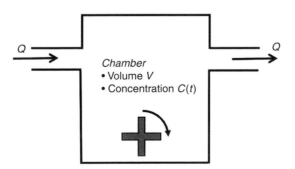

$$\bar{t} = \frac{\int_0^\infty tC(t)dt}{\int_0^\infty C(t)dt}$$

(a) Define the standard deviation of the transit time.

(b) Consider a well-mixed fluid chamber of fixed volume V into which fluid is delivered through one port and removed through a second port, both at a flow rate Q. Find the mean chamber transit time and the standard deviation of the transit time for the case in which a bolus of tracer (of original concentration C_0 in a volume V_0) is delivered in the chamber's inlet stream. The volume V_0 can be assumed to be much smaller than V.

13.21. Heat transfer to biological tissues is complicated by the presence of blood vessels, since flowing blood delivers and/or removes heat from the tissue region. We wish to derive a modified form of the unsteady-heat-conduction equation that includes the effect of heat convection in blood as a single additional term.

(a) Consider a differential element of tissue that is perfused with arterial blood at a rate of ω (cm^3 of blood per cm^3 of tissue per second) and allow this blood to have a temperature of T_b. The differential element is tiny, but large enough that the temperature of blood leaving the element (venous blood) is the same as the tissue temperature of the element. Find this modified form of the heat-conduction equation, which we call the "bioheat" equation.

(b) Assume that a small spherical region ($R = 2$ cm) of the body is cooled to a temperature of 5 °C. When the device used to cool the tissue is removed, roughly estimate how long it will take this tissue to return to within 0.5 °C of normal body temperature (you may ignore the effects of conduction in your analysis). Use a value of $\omega = 0.0028$ s^{-1}. You may use the properties of water to characterize the properties of the tissue and the blood.

14 Concentration and thermal boundary layers

(7 concentration problems; 2 thermal problems)

14.1. In a microfluidic device used to subject cells to a concentration gradient of a growth factor G, two streams of fluid enter at one end, flow through a channel of rectangular cross-section, and exit at the other end (see the sketch below). As soon as the two streams come into contact with one another (at $x = 0$), they begin to diffuse into each other, smearing the initially distinct surface separating them at the entrance.

Assuming that the two streams of fluid move at the same <u>uniform</u> velocity v_x, and that factor G diffuses from stream B into stream A with a diffusivity D_G, obtain an <u>approximate</u> expression for the distance over which a cross-stream gradient exists as a function of distance along the channel, $\delta(x)$. Be sure to explain your reasoning.

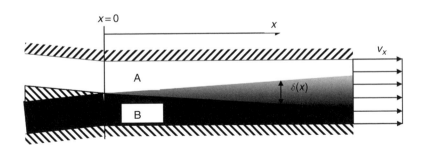

14.2. Dry air flows over a 1-m-long flat pan containing water that is evaporating. The system is isothermal. The free-stream velocity of the air is $V_\infty = 2$ m/s and the air's kinematic viscosity is 1.55×10^{-5} m^2/s. We define L^* to be the axial location such that half of the pan's total mass transfer (water to air) occurs over the range $0 \leq x \leq L^*$ and the other half of the total mass transfer occurs over the range $L^* \leq x \leq L$. What is L^*?

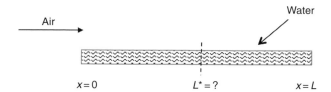

Air

Water

$x = 0$ $L^* = ?$ $x = L$

14.3. Stents are used to maintain the patency of occluded blood vessels (i.e. to prop them open) after angioplasty. However, cells in the vessel wall can sometimes continue to proliferate and secrete extracellular material, leading to re-occlusion of the vessel. One solution to this problem is to use stents that release into the blood vessel wall drugs that inhibit this cellular proliferation. The drug to be used has a diffusion coefficient in tissue of $D_{wall} = 1 \times 10^{-7}$ cm^2/s and a diffusion constant in the blood of $D_{blood} = 3 \times 10^{-7}$ cm^2/s.

We wish to consider one potential design of this system. The stent can be treated as a thin porous, cylindrical shell (of length $L = 2$ cm, inner radius $R - T = 0.2$ cm, and thickness $T = 0.01$ cm) that is loaded with the drug at an original concentration of $C_s(t = 0) = C_0 = 5$ mg/cm^3. This drug is released from the porous shell such that the concentration of drug immediately adjacent to both the inner and outer radius of this shell is $\alpha C_s(t)$, where $C_s(t)$ is the drug concentration in the stent (which is assumed to be spatially uniform) and $\alpha = 3 \times 10^{-5}$.

The wall of the blood vessel also has an inner radius of $R = 0.2$ cm and a wall thickness of $\delta = 0.07$ cm, which is much larger than T; for simplicity we will treat δ as being much smaller than R. The drug is removed from the outer surface of the blood vessel ($r = R + \delta$) at a rate (per unit surface area) of $\beta C(r = R + \delta)$ with $\beta = 2.5 \times 10^{-6}$ cm/s; that is, the removal rate is proportional to the concentration of drug at the outer surface of the blood vessel. The drug saturates receptors on cells in the wall at a very low concentration, and thus, while pharmacologically significant, the binding of drug to mural cells is not important in considering the overall kinetics of drug transport across the artery wall.

(a) After the initial placement of the stent, approximately how long does it take before the entire thickness of the blood vessel wall is exposed to a significant quantity of the drug.

(b) Now assume that a long time has passed such that the concentration of drug in the blood vessel wall is quasi-steady, that is $C(r, t)$ is proportional to $C_s(t)$. Furthermore, since $\delta \ll R$, you may assume that the concentration profile in the blood vessel wall is linear. Find the concentration of drug at the outer surface of the blood vessel as a function of $C_s(t)$.

(c) While some drug is being removed from the stent by diffusion of the drug into the blood vessel wall, most of the drug is lost into the blood flow passing through the vessel into which the stent is placed. Assuming a blood flow rate of 80 ml/min through the blood vessel, roughly estimate how long this stent will continue to release drug into the tissue. Blood has a density of 1.05 g/cm^3 and a viscosity of 0.035 g/cm per s.

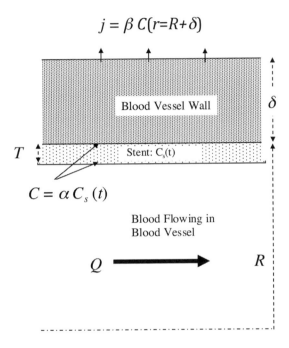

$$j = \beta\,C(r=R+\delta)$$

14.4. An experiment is being conducted to study signaling between two types of cells. Cell type A has been grown to confluence on the upper surface of a rectangular chamber, while cell type B has been grown to confluence on the lower surface of this chamber (see the figure overleaf). Cell type A produces a protein that it secretes into the medium below the cell. Cell type B binds this protein from the medium. The diffusion coefficient of this protein in the medium is 1×10^{-7} cm^2/s. The separation between the two layers of cells is $s = 200$ μm, the length of the chamber is $L = 4$ mm, and the width of the chamber is $w = 1$ cm. You may assume that the concentration of protein at the surface of the cells of type B is effectively zero, since these cells bind the protein nearly instantaneously when it arrives at their surface. The fluid has a density of 1 g/ml and a viscosity of 0.01 g/ml per s. Assume that a steady state pertains.

(a) We would like to perfuse medium through the system at flow rate Q to provide oxygen to the cells, but we want to make sure that this flow does not disrupt the signaling between the two cell layers. Roughly estimate the maximum flow rate, Q_1, at which there is negligible disruption of this diffusional signaling between the cell layers.

(b) Consider this very low flow rate Q_1 for which the transport of protein from the upper to the lower surface is entirely by diffusion and unaffected by the flow. At the exit of the chamber, the flow is split into two streams at exactly the midpoint of the channel. The upper stream is collected and the protein concentration in this fluid is measured to be 1 mg/ml. Give an expression (in terms of known quantities) for the concentration of protein in the media immediately adjacent to the cells of type A.

(c) Binding of the secreted protein by cell type B is hypothesized to cause a change in the activity of these cells. To confirm this, we would like to perform a controlled experiment in which some of the cells of type B are exposed to this protein while others are not. Roughly estimate a flow rate Q_2 passing through this chamber that causes the cells in the upstream half of the chamber ($x < 2$ mm) to not be exposed to the secreted protein, while the cells in the downstream half of the chamber ($x > 2$ mm) will be exposed.

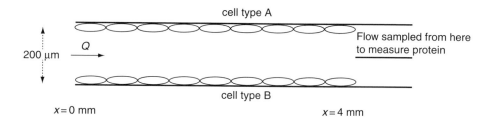

14.5. Cells are cultured on a flat cover slip in a large flow chamber. Culture medium, supplemented by 0.3 ng/ml connective tissue growth factor (CTGF), flows over the cells at a velocity of 1.5 cm/s. After 8 days the cover slip is removed from the chamber and the thickness of the basement membrane produced by the cells, T_{BM}, is measured and found to follow the relationship

$$T_{BM} = A_1 x^{-b}$$

with $b = 0.23$ and $A_1 = 0.85$ µm cm$^{0.23}$ in the region 3 cm $\leq x \leq 8$ cm, where x is as shown in the figure.

(a) For the region of interest ($3 \text{ cm} \leq x \leq 8 \text{ cm}$), is the boundary layer laminar or turbulent? Take the kinematic viscosity of the culture medium at 37 °C to be $7 \times 10^{-3} \text{ cm}^2/\text{s}$.

(b) We hypothesize that CTGF stimulates the production of basement membrane by cells. Define g_{BM} to be the local <u>rate</u> of deposition of basement membrane (thickness per unit time, a constant at any location) and j to be the local flux (mass per area unit time) of CTGF to the cells. Show that the above measurements of basement-membrane thickness are consistent with a relationship of the form $g_{BM} = A_2 j^{2b}$, where A_2 is a constant. You may assume that CTGF binds rapidly and irreversibly to cultured cells, and that there is no basement membrane present when cells are first plated onto the cover slip.

(c) Compute the value of A_2. Take the diffusion coefficient of CTGF in culture medium to be $3 \times 10^{-6} \text{ cm}^2/\text{s}$. (Be careful: the units are nasty here.)

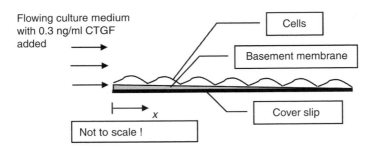

Flowing culture medium with 0.3 ng/ml CTGF added

Cells

Basement membrane

Cover slip

x

Not to scale !

14.6. An investigator who is studying a very small fish has discovered that this fish exudes a chemical from the front of its body, near its gills (see the diagram overleaf). This chemical appears to be very noxious, and has a diffusivity in water of $D = 1 \times 10^{-5} \text{ cm}^2/\text{s}$. The hypothesis is that, as the fish swims along, this chemical is released, diffuses away from the body of the fish, and dissuades other larger fish from attacking this small fish. The water in which the fish swims is at a temperature of 20 °C.

We would like to evaluate this hypothesis. We will model the fish as a two-sided flat plate of length 4 cm and height 0.5 cm, with the chemical being released from the front of the plate. This small fish swims at an average speed of 10 cm/s.

(a) If a predator attacked the fish from the side, what is the maximum distance from the fish at which a predator would detect the noxious agent?

(b) Is the hypothesis reasonable?

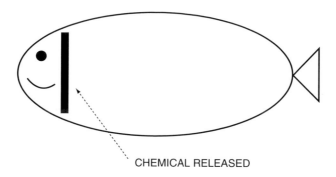

CHEMICAL RELEASED

14.7. Consider the situation depicted in the figure below, in which fluid flows over a cell monolayer that begins at $x = 0$. The fluid velocity can be approximated as linear in the region close to the monolayer, which is described by

$$v_x = \dot{\gamma} y$$

A protein is secreted by the cells, and diffuses upward at the same time as it is convected downstream by the velocity profile. You may assume that the velocity profile does not change with distance x, that $v_y = v_z = 0$, and that a steady-state solution exists. The given quantities are the shear rate, $\dot{\gamma}$, the protein diffusion coefficient, D, and the concentration of protein at the cell layer, C_0, which is independent of x.

(a) Find the reduced form of the transport equation and boundary conditions appropriate for this situation.
(b) Obtain a scaling relationship for the dependence of the boundary-layer thickness, δ, on the given parameters of the problem.
(c) Use your scaling relation to determine an appropriate similarity variable, η, for this problem. Show that the transport equation and boundary conditions conform to a similarity solution.
(d) Find the solution to the similarity equation and plot C/C_0 vs. η.
(e) Obtain an expression for the flux of protein from the cell surface, as a function of x.

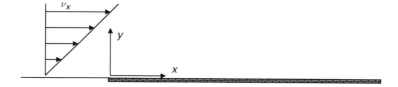

14.8. Casinos are frequently open all night long. In some places, they don't even have front doors. Instead of a door, they use a flow of warm air (in the winter) from an opening in the ceiling that is collected at the floor. Assuming that the air flows uniformly (from ceiling to floor) in a space of width 3 m, height 5 m, and thickness 1 m, make a rough estimate of the air flow rate necessary in order to keep the region of the casino near the entrance from being cold during the winter. Let the temperature at the doorway be 20 °C. Solve assuming both laminar and turbulent flow conditions. For turbulent flow (due to outside wind and people moving in and out of the doorway), use a value for the effective thermal diffusivity of 10 m^2/s. Decide which answer better models the situation.

14.9. On cold winter days, it is necessary to heat up the car before driving, especially to warm up the windshield glass so that it does not fog up and obscure vision. Consider a very cold day such that the windshield glass (of thermal conductivity $k_{glass} = 1.0$ W/m per K, density $\rho_{glass} = 2500$ kg/m^3, and heat capacity $C_{glass} = 840$ J/kg per K) is at a temperature of –10 °F. Air has a density of $\rho_a = 1.34$ kg/m^3, a viscosity of $\mu_a = 1.7 \times 10^{-5}$ kg/m per s, a heat capacity of $C_a = 1000$ J/kg per K, and a thermal conductivity of $k_a = 0.024$ W/m per K. (Note that 1 W = 1 J/s.)

The windshield is 0.7 cm thick and has a total height of 60 cm; the width of the windshield is 170 cm. Assume that the location at which your eyes look out of the window is 30 cm from the bottom.

When turning on the defroster, let the temperature of the air blowing onto the inside of the windshield be 90 °F, and let the velocity of this air be 5 m/s. Since the car is not moving and the air outside the car is stationary, you may assume that the window is essentially insulated on its outside surface.

(a) Plot the heat-transfer coefficient (h) from the blowing air to the windshield as a function of distance from the bottom of the windshield ($x = 0$).

(b) Estimate how long it will take until the temperature of the windshield at eye level and below is greater than 32 °F (the better your estimate, the better your score).

(c) Now consider that a new "super glass" (made of industrial diamonds) that has a very high thermal conductivity ($k = 1200$ W/m per K), with its other properties the same as those of regular glass, has been developed. Determine how long it will take until the temperature of this window is everywhere greater than 32 °F.

15 Mass and heat transfer coefficients

(11 mass-transfer problems; 3 heat-transfer problems)

15.1. In a blood oxygenator, the blood spends approximately 2 s passing through the device. Estimate a minimum value for h_m, the mass transfer coefficient characterizing oxygen transport from the plasma to the inside of a red blood cell (RBC), such that the RBCs are completely (i.e. >99%) oxygenated before leaving the oxygenator (100% oxygenated refers to the maximum oxygen loading the cells can achieve in this oxygenator if the RBCs were left in the oxygenator for a very long time). You may assume that the RBCs entering the device are 50% oxygenated. Let the volume of each RBC be 98 μm^3 and its surface area be 130 μm^2. The diffusion coefficient of oxygen both in plasma and inside of the cell can be taken as 2×10^{-5} cm^2/s.

15.2. A porous block attached to an air line emits tiny air bubbles (of diameter 0.15 mm, 21% oxygen) at the bottom of a fish tank filled with water at 25 °C. The absolute pressure in the bubbles at the bottom of the tank is 1.07×10^6 g/cm per s^2 when they are released. They reach their terminal upward velocity almost instantly, since they enter the tank at nearly this velocity. Find the rate of oxygen transfer from one of these bubbles to the water. You may neglect the concentration of oxygen already in the water. The diffusion coefficient of oxygen in water is 2×10^{-5} cm^2/s.

15.3. An experimental study involves lining the inside of microtubes (of radius 30 μm) with a monolayer of cells that produces a compound of interest. We are concerned with making sure that CO_2 produced by these cells is adequately removed.

The cells on the inside of the microtubes produce CO_2 at a rate of 6×10^{-7} g/cm^2 per s (this is the rate per unit surface area of the tube, not the total rate). The perfusion medium (with properties similar to those of saline) entering the tube is essentially free of CO_2. The length of each of the microtubes is 0.3 cm. What minimum flow rate must pass through each tube to ensure that the maximum level of CO_2 to which any cell is exposed is less than 1×10^{-4} g/ml?

The diffusion coefficient of CO_2 in the medium is 2×10^{-5} cm^2/s. The velocity and concentration profiles may be assumed to be fully developed. You may neglect the thickness of the cells in your calculation of the tube radius. You may also neglect axial diffusion, but should justify this assumption.

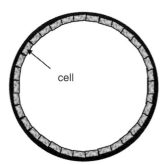

cell

15.4. Endothelial cells are grown on the inside surface of hollow fibers with radius 100 μm ($r = R$) and length 150 cm. The cells contain an enzyme that converts a toxin A into a harmless species at a rate that is proportional to the perfused surface area and to the toxin concentration at the cell surface. Thus, $\hat{j}$, the detoxification rate per unit area of the fiber wall, is

$$\hat{j}(x) = k'C(x, r = R)$$

where k' is a rate constant and C is the concentration of toxin.

Blood flow is delivered to each fiber at a rate of 60 μl/min. The diffusion coefficient of the toxin in the blood is 5×10^{-7} cm^2/s. The system is at a temperature of 37 °C.

Consider two cases: (i) $k' = 2.5 \times 10^{-6}$ cm/s and (ii) $k' = 2 \times 10^{-3}$ cm/s.

(a) Find a criterion, <u>for this problem</u>, to determine whether this reaction is reaction-rate-limited or diffusion-limited at the wall in each case.

(b) If the inlet concentration of toxin in the blood is 0.5 mm, find the toxin concentration at the exit of each fiber for the above two values of k'. Justify any assumptions you make.

15.5. Consider a long tube (1 mm in diameter) through which a solution (with $\mu = 0.01$ g/cm per s and $\rho = 1$ g/cm^3) is flowing. The tube wall is sufficiently porous to allow oxygen transport into the solution, and the oxygen concentration at the wall is held constant at 5.6×10^{-6} g/ml. The diffusivity of oxygen in the solution is 2×10^{-5} cm^2/s. The pressure drop driving the flow is 5 mm Hg, and you may assume that the velocity and concentration profiles in the tube are fully developed.

(a) First assume that the solution is cell-free, so there is no oxygen uptake by cells in the solution. Assume that the solution entering the tube is oxygen-free. How long must the tube be in order for the average oxygen concentration, $\overline{C}$, in the solution at the exit of the tube to be 1.4×10^{-6} g/ml?

(b) Now assume that the solution contains a homogeneous suspension of cells and that the oxygen-consumption rate of these cells (per unit volume of solution) is 2.75×10^{-8} g/ml per s. Consider a location far enough downstream from the inlet that $d\overline{C}/dx = 0$. Find the Sherwood number for this case, and find the average oxygen concentration in the flowing solution. (Hint: the Sherwood number is not the same as in part (a).)

15.6. Cells completely cover the inner surface of a cylindrical tube 2 mm in diameter and 6 cm long. Culture medium (with kinematic viscosity $v = 0.015$ cm^2/s) flows through the tube with a mean velocity of $V = 0.075$ cm/s. The area of each cell is 450 μm^2, and each cell produces a peptide at a constant rate of 0.005 ng/s. The peptide enters the flowing medium, where its diffusion coefficient is 5×10^{-7} cm^2/s. Assuming that there is no peptide in the culture medium when it enters the tube, compute the average and surface concentrations of the peptide at the outlet of the tube.

The graph (from [13]) on the next page shows heat-transfer data that you might find useful. Here Nu_{loc} is the local (as opposed to average) Nusselt number (which is based on the tube diameter), α is the thermal diffusivity, z is the axial distance along the tube or slit, R is the tube radius, B is the slit separation, and $\langle v_z \rangle$ is the average fluid velocity passing through the slit or tube. You will have to "translate" this graph from heat to mass transfer for use in this question.

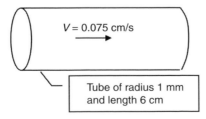

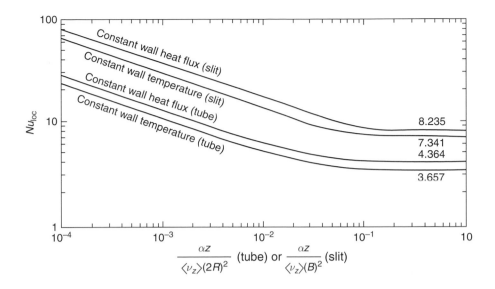

15.7. In a bioreactor, cells and extracellular matrix are cast in cylindrical rods of radius $S = 200$ μm and length $L = 2$ cm (see the figure below). Nutrients are brought to the cells by a flow that passes around these rods, and waste products are carried away. We are interested in making sure that the CO_2 is adequately removed.

Let the rate of CO_2 production per unit volume in each cylindrical rod be $\alpha = 5 \times 10^{-7}$ mol/ml per h. Let the velocity of the saline ($\rho = 1$ g/ml; $\mu = 0.01$ g/cm per s) passing around these rods be $V = 1$ cm/s. The diffusion coefficient of CO_2 in the rod

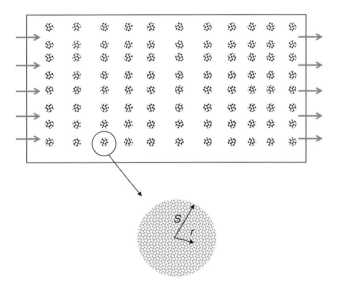

is $D_r = 1 \times 10^{-5}$ cm^2/s, while the diffusion coefficient of CO_2 in the saline is $D_s = 2 \times 10^{-5}$ cm^2/s. Assume steady-state conditions. You may assume that the concentration of CO_2 in the saline far from a cell (C_∞) is negligible, and that the flow field around each cylinder is essentially the same as if it were an isolated cylinder.

(a) Find $C(r)$, the concentration distribution in one of these rods (see the enlargement of one rod shown below the main part of the figure).

(b) Calculate the peak concentration of CO_2 (at $r = 0$) inside of one of these rods.

15.8. A cylindrical bioreactor of diameter 4 cm is designed to produce recombinant protein. Cells in a suspension culture (with a density of 10^4 cells/ml) produce 6×10^{-22} mol/h per cell of protein. The cell chamber (the shaded part of the diagram) is well stirred such that the concentration of the produced protein is everywhere constant in the chamber, outside of the central tube.

The protein diffuses through a very thin porous wall of a central tube (there is no resistance to transport through this thin wall) and is collected by culture medium

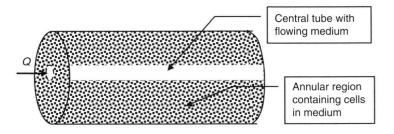

Central tube with flowing medium

Q

Annular region containing cells in medium

flowing through this tube at $Q = 4 \times 10^{-6}$ ml/s. The central tube has an inner diameter of 2 mm and a length 10 cm. The protein diffusivity in the flowing medium is 3×10^{-8} cm^2/s. Note that the protein is not well stirred in this central tube.

Determine the average protein concentration in the fluid within the annular region containing the cells. You can neglect entrance effects, and thus assume a constant mass-transfer coefficient along the length of the tube. Assume that a steady state has been attained. The culture medium has a density of 1 g/cm^3 and a viscosity of 0.01 g/cm per s. State and justify any assumptions you make.

15.9. Rectangular microchannels are to be micro-machined onto a chip to be used for culturing liver cells in a matrix. These channels have a height of 60 μm and a width of $W = 500$ μm. Our goal is to determine how long these channels can be while ensuring that all of the cells receive an adequate supply of oxygen.

The bottom 50 μm of each channel is to be filled with a tissue mixture that includes both extracellular matrix and liver cells. The top 10 μm of each channel is left free, so fluid can flow through this narrow channel and carry oxygen and nutrients to the cells, and carry away waste products. (Note that the tissue layer will then have fluid both above it and below it, since the bottom of each channel is adjacent to the next channel.)

Let the entering perfusion fluid have an oxygen content of $C_0 = 5.6 \times 10^{-5}$ g/ml. The fluid has the same transport properties as water. The tissue has an oxygen-consumption rate (per unit volume) of 1.1×10^{-4} g/ml per s, and the diffusion coefficient of the oxygen through the tissue (and through the perfusion fluid) is 2×10^{-5} cm^2/s. The perfusion fluid is supplied to the entrance of the microchannel at a pressure of 200 mm Hg (relative to atmospheric pressure), and exits the channel at approximately atmospheric pressure. The temperature everywhere is 37 °C.

What is the maximum length of these channels such that all of the cells receive oxygen? You may assume that steady-state conditions pertain and that the velocity and concentration profiles are all fully developed.

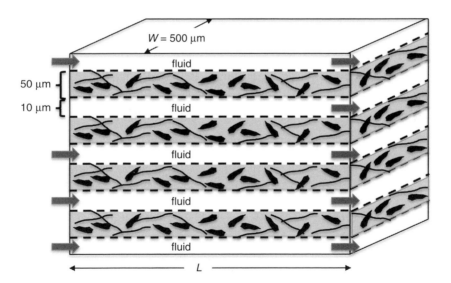

15.10. An artificial kidney uses porous hollow fibers to purify blood. Blood containing urea flows through the fibers and the urea diffuses out, through the porous fiber walls. Typically, tens of thousands of such fibers are used in an artificial kidney. We would like to determine the fraction of the urea removed as the blood flows through one such fiber.

Consider a fiber of radius $R = 100$ μm and length $L = 10$ cm with a flow rate of blood (viscosity 0.03 g/cm per s and density of 1.06 g/ml) through this fiber of $Q_0 = 10$ μl/min. Let the flux of urea (j_w) out through the fiber wall be

$$j_w = PC_w$$

where $P = 1.3 \times 10^{-3}$ cm/s is the permeability of the fiber wall to urea, and $C_w(x)$ is the concentration of urea at the wall of the fiber ($r = R$) at axial location x ($0 < x < L$). The diffusion coefficient of urea in the blood is 1×10^{-5} cm^2/s. Because saline also leaks through the porous wall of this fiber, the flow rate decreases along the length of the tube. The leakage flow through the porous wall has a magnitude of $V_w = 0.25$ cm^3/h per cm^2 surface area of fiber. You can neglect the urea that is carried through the tube wall by this leakage flow.

The Sherwood number for the transfer of urea from the flow in the tube (mean concentration $\overline{C}$) to the wall (concentration C_w) follows this relationship:

$$Sh \equiv \frac{h_m R}{D} = 1.58 + 2.5 \frac{V_w R}{D}$$

where h_m is defined by the expression $j = h_m(\overline{C} - C_w)$ and j is the flux to the wall. Assume steady-state conditions.

(a) Find an expression for $d\overline{C}/dx$ in the hollow fiber in terms of parameters given above.

(b) Find the fraction of urea that is removed as blood flows through this fiber (by comparing blood entering with blood leaving).

(c) Justify the assumption that one can neglect the urea that is carried through the tube wall by the leakage flow.

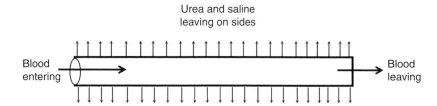

15.11. A design of a human gill has been proposed using a bed of parallel, hollow fibers made of membranes with a very high permeability to oxygen. Blood (at 37 °C) flows over these fibers (in cross-flow) at a mean velocity of 1 cm/s, while saline (from the ocean at 20 °C) passes through them at an average velocity of 8 cm/s. To support a 70-kg human, Yang and Cussler [14, 15] determined that the gill would have to extract up to 2500 ml/min of oxygen (at atmospheric pressure) from the seawater.

The outer diameter of each fiber is 0.4 mm, its wall thickness is 30 μm, and its length is 15 cm. The fibers are made of microporous polypropylene with a pore size of 30 nm. Pores cover 33% of the fiber surface and are filled with physiologic saline, so that the oxygen diffuses through these pores from the seawater inside the fibers to the blood outside the fibers. The solid (non-porous) part of the polypropylene can be assumed to be impermeable to oxygen.

The Sherwood number for mass transfer from the surface of the hollow fibers to the blood flowing over these fibers (perpendicular to the axes of the parallel fibers) is

$$Sh = 1.4(Re\ Sc)^{0.33}$$

where the velocity of the flow used in this equation is the average velocity of blood passing over the fibers, the Reynolds number Re is based on the outer diameter of the fibers, and Sc is the Schmidt number for oxygen in blood.

The concentration of oxygen in the incoming saline is 1.5×10^{-6} mol/cm^3. You may assume that the effective concentration of oxygen in the blood is always much lower than the concentration in the saline since the oxygen is rapidly bound to hemoglobin in the red blood cells as soon as the oxygen enters the blood.

The diffusion coefficient of oxygen in blood is 1.5×10^{-5} cm^2/s, and that in saline is 3×10^{-5} cm^2/s. Explain and justify any assumptions that you make.

(a) Determine a mass-transfer coefficient (U) that allows the determination of the flux (j) of oxygen across the membrane at any axial location x, where $j(x) = UC(x)$ and $C(x)$ is the average concentration of oxygen inside the fiber at axial location x. (Note that the unbound concentration of oxygen in the blood outside the fiber is assumed to be much lower than this.)

(b) Determine the total area of hollow fiber membrane that would be necessary in order for this system to support a person.

(c) Explain why the system would be poorly designed if the blood were to pass through the fibers while the saline passed over the fibers.

15.12. A naked adult falls into water at a temperature of 2 °C. The person treads water to maintain their position against a current of 0.5 m/s. Water at 2 °C has a thermal conductivity of 0.57 W/m per K, a Prandtl number of 12.2, and a kinematic viscosity of 0.016 cm^2/s. You may neglect the influence of treading water on the heat transfer process.

(a)   Model the person as a cylinder with a diameter of 30.5 cm, a height of 1.73 m, and a surface area of 1.8 m². Assume that there is a central core region of radius 10 cm whose temperature is maintained at 37 °C. The tissue surrounding this central core has a thermal conductivity of 0.41 W/m per K, and the blood circulation and heat generation in this surrounding tissue can be neglected. Find the rate of heat loss from the person and their skin temperature. Assume steady-state conditions.

(b)   Now have the same person wearing a wet suit made of 7-mm-thick neoprene, which insulates the skin by trapping nitrogen bubbles in the foam. The thermal conductivity of this neoprene foam is 0.054 W/m per K. Find the steady-state rate of heat loss from the person and their skin temperature, under these conditions.

15.13. Fluid velocity can be measured using a "hot-wire anemometer" in which a wire is placed into a flow and heated with an electrical current. If the temperature of the fluid stream is known, and the temperature of the wire and the current delivered to it are measured, the velocity of the fluid can be deduced. Such an anemometer can be used to measure air velocity in a spirometer, a device used to measure the airflow in a forced exhalation.

Let a wire 0.2 mm in diameter be placed in an airflow. The wire is heated by electrical current and maintains a temperature of 40 °C while air at 37 °C flows over it. Under these conditions, the wire dissipates 1 W/m of heat. How fast is the air flowing?

15.14. Operating-room heat exchangers can cool blood (bypassed from the patient) and thereby cool the patient to slow physiologic processes and thus allow longer surgical times. Consider a procedure whereby the blood (of density 1.05 g/ml, viscosity 3.5 g/cm per s, thermal conductivity 0.5 W/m per °C, and heat capacity 3.6 kJ/kg per °C) flows through coiled tubes in a heat exchanger with a flow rate in each small tube of 0.2 ml/s. The coiled tubes are made of Teflon (of thermal conductivity 0.23 W/m per °C) with an inner diameter of 1.0 mm and an outer diameter of 1.3 mm (you can ignore the effect of the coiling on the internal flow of the blood). They are surrounded by an ice-and-water bath that is agitated with a mixer to generate an average heat-transfer coefficient at the outer surface of the coil of 500 W/m² per °C. How long should each tube be in order to cool the blood from an average temperature of 37 °C to 32 °C?

You may assume that the inside of the Teflon tube is at a relatively constant temperature along its length. Assume the velocity and temperature profiles to be fully developed, and you may also neglect changes in the properties of the blood as it is cooled.

16 Osmotic pressure

(6 problems)

16.1. Consider a membrane of thickness 10 μm that has a number of tiny cylindrical pores (of radius 10 nm) passing through it. The density of pores in the membrane is such that the porosity (fractions of water-filled space) of the membrane is 0.1%.

(a) Find the hydraulic conductivity (L_p, flow rate per unit area per unit pressure drop) of this membrane.

(b) Consider a 4 mM solution of a large protein on one side of this membrane and physiologic saline on the other, with the same pressure on both sides of the membrane. Assume that the protein is sufficiently large that it cannot pass through the membrane and that van 't Hoff's law holds for this solute. Calculate the initial flow rate of saline through a membrane of area 5 cm^2 at a temperature of 300 K.

16.2. The graph shown in the figure overleaf is adapted from a 1927 paper [16] in which Landis proved the existence of Starling's phenomenon by occluding capillaries. The ordinate is the volume of fluid leaking out of (or re-entering) the capillary per unit capillary wall area, j. Although it is not precisely true, for the purposes of this question you may assume that the reflection coefficient of this capillary wall to plasma proteins is unity.

(a) Assuming that $p - \Pi$ for the interstitium is –5 cm H_2O, estimate the plasma osmotic pressure (Π) from the figure. Note that the plasma proteins are the main species influencing the osmotic pressure difference across the capillary wall.

(b) Estimate the filtration coefficient L_p for this capillary.

(c) Consider a capillary 0.05 cm long of diameter 8 μm, for which the arteriolar and venular luminal pressures are 25 and 5 cm H_2O, respectively. Assume that L_p and Π are constant and that the pressure drop varies linearly along the capillary. What is the net rate of fluid loss (gain) from the capillary?

In the above analysis, we assumed that the capillary plasma protein osmotic pressure Π_{cap} did not change with axial position within the capillary, x. Strictly speaking, this is not true, since leakage of saline from the capillary increases the effective protein concentration in the capillary, and hence increases the osmotic pressure. In parts (d)–(f), we examine the validity of the assumption of constant osmotic pressure in the vessel.

(d)   Using the data given above, find the balance point for the capillary, i.e. the location x where there is no net transport of fluid to or from the tissue.

(e)   How much fluid is lost per unit time from the capillary between the inlet and the balance point, assuming that Π_{cap} is constant?

(f)   The total flow rate entering the capillary is $4.2 \times 10^4 \ \mu m^3/s$, consisting of 42% red blood cells (RBCs), 4% plasma proteins, and 54% saline (by volume). What is the percentage change in protein osmotic pressure at the balance point (referenced to the protein osmotic pressure at the inlet)? Assume that van 't Hoff's law holds, and that there is no protein or RBC leakage through the capillary wall. Is our assumption of an approximately constant Π_{cap} a valid one? From [2].

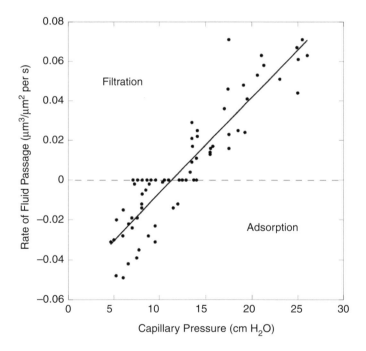

16.3. A physiologic saline solution contains two proteins, one small that has a molecular radius of 1 nm, and the other quite large with a radius of 5 nm. The concentrations of the small and large proteins (P_S and P_L) in this solution are 4 mM and 1 mM, respectively. The solution is at a temperature of 25 °C, and has the same viscosity and density as water. We wish to remove the small protein from the solution while retaining the larger protein.

To do this, we will use a dialysis membrane with cylindrical pores that have a radius of 4 nm and a length of 100 nm; the porosity (the volume of pores divided by the volume of membrane) of the membrane is 25%. Thus the small molecules pass easily through the membrane but the large molecules are completely rejected. The idea is to put this protein solution into a highly flexible bag made of this membrane and then put a pure saline solution outside the bag. The small proteins will diffuse out through the membrane eventually, leaving a solution with only large proteins on the inside of the bag. You may assume that the solutions both inside and outside the bag are well stirred.

Our concern is that the difference in osmotic pressure on the two sides of the membrane will generate a flow of fluid into the bag and prevent the small protein from diffusing out. The diffusion coefficient of the small protein through the membrane is 5×10^{-6} cm^2/s.

We want to model the transport through one of the pores in the membrane.

(a) Find the flow rate entering each pore due to the osmotic pressure difference when the dialysis bag is first placed into the saline solution. You may assume that the pressure of the fluid is the same on both sides of the membrane.

(b) Determine whether the flow of saline into the bag will appreciably slow the diffusion of the small protein out of the bag.

(c) Find an equivalent h that characterizes the mass-transfer rate of P_S per unit area of membrane (j) out of the bag, defined by $j = h(C_i - C_o)$, where C_i is the concentration of the small protein inside the bag and C_o is the concentration of the small protein outside the bag at any particular point in time.

16.4. A membrane of hydraulic permeability L_p and area A_m separates two chambers, each of volume V. At time $t = 0$, m_1 moles of solute are added to chamber 1 and m_2 moles are added to chamber 2, where $m_2 > m_1$. You may assume that solute mixes and dissolves in each chamber very rapidly, that the membrane is impermeable to the solute, and that the densities of the resulting two solutions are approximately equal to ρ. Attached to each chamber is a riser tube (see the figure overleaf) of cross-sectional area A_1 (chamber 1) or A_2 (chamber 2), where $A_2 \ll A_1$. At $t = 0$ the fluid levels in the two tubes are equal, as shown. You may assume that $V \gg A_2 h(t)$ for all time.

What is the height of solution in tube 2 as a function of time, i.e. what is $h_2(t)$? Take the $h_2 = 0$ reference point as shown in the figure. State relevant assumptions. From [2].

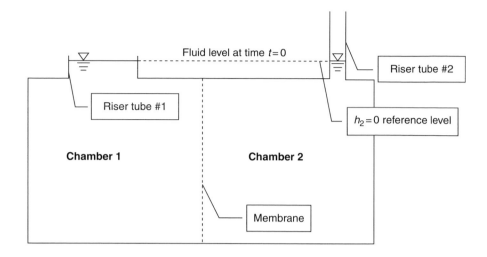

16.5. In certain applications, blood is first diluted and then later needs to be concentrated to its original concentration. The latter step can be done with a dialyser such as that shown in the figure above. The dialysate solution has glucose added to it so that it is hypertonic (has an osmotic pressure greater than that of the blood). This causes water to move into the dialysate, even though the pressure in the blood is equal to that in the dialysate.

Let $Q(x)$ be the volume rate of blood flow, $C(x)$ the molar concentration of osmotically active components in the blood, and $C_d(x)$ the molar concentration of osmotically active substances in the dialysate. Let the depth of the dialyser into the page be D. We will assume that *only* water can cross the membrane. We will also assume that the blood and the dialysate obey van 't Hoff's law for osmotic pressure, and let R be the ideal-gas constant and T the temperature.

(a)   Let $Q(x = 0) = Q_0$ and $C(x=0)=C_0$. Find $C(x)$ as a function of $Q(x)$.

(b)   Let L_p be the permeability (flow rate per unit area per unit osmotic pressure difference) of the membrane separating the blood from the glucose solution. Find $dQ(x)/dx$ in terms of $C(x)$ and $C_d(x)$.

(c)   Find a differential equation for $C(x)$ in terms of known quantities and $C_d(x)$. Note that $Q(x)$ is not a known quantity.

(d)   If the flow rate of the dialysate is large, the concentration of glucose in the dialysate can be considered constant. Furthermore, in some situations, $C_d(x) \gg C(x)$ (molar concentration). Making this assumption, solve the differential equation for $C(x)$.

(e)   If $Q_0 = 250$ ml/min, $C_0 = 0.05$ mol/l, $D = 10$ cm, and $C_d = 0.5$ mol/l, find the necessary length (L) of the dialyser such that $C(L) = 0.2$ mol/l (you may

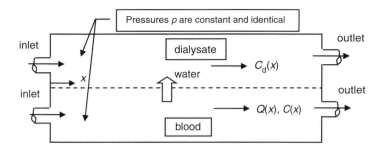

assume that $C_d(x) \gg C(x)$). Here L_p is 1×10^{-8} cm/s per Pa, the temperature is 310 K, and the universal gas constant R is 8.314 J/mol per K (modified from Ethier and Simmons [2]).

16.6. Red blood cells (RBCs) are normally in osmotic equilibrium with the surrounding plasma. However, if they are placed in a hypotonic solution (i.e. one having lower than physiologic osmotic pressure), they will swell, since the cell membrane is effectively impermeable to ions but allows the water to pass through.

Consider a cell of initial internal volume $V_i = 98$ μm^3, and initial surface area $A_i = 130$ μm^2 having initial internal total ionic concentration $C_i = 300$ mM. The RBC membrane allows no ions to pass and has a water permeability of $L_p = 1 \times 10^{-11}$ cm^2 s/g (flow rate per unit membrane area per unit transmembrane pressure difference).

At $t = 0$, the cell is placed in a very large hypotonic bathing solution having total ionic concentration $C_o < C_i$. Assume that van 't Hoff's law holds, namely $\Pi = RTC$. Furthermore, assume that as an RBC swells, its internal pressure (P) increases with increasing surface area (A) as $dP/dA = (300$ dyne/cm$)/V_c$, where V_c is the cell volume. The RBC membranes are stiff and relatively inextensible. Assume that the cell will rupture if the cell membrane area is stretched by more than 6%. We are interested in determining by how much the volume of this cell can increase before it bursts.

You may assume that the pressures inside and outside of the cell are equal when the cell is placed into the hypotonic bath at room temperature (298 K).

(a) Draw a sequence of events showing how the RBC changes its size and shape as it expands. You may assume that, as the volume of the RBC increases, its surface area remains constant until its shape is spherical. Further volume increases lead to increases in surface area.

(b) Predict the lowest value of C_o that the cell can tolerate without bursting.

(c) Estimate how much time it will take for an RBC to burst when placed into distilled water. To make this estimate, you may ignore the changing internal pressure (P) and surface area (A) of the RBC as it swells (modified from Ethier and Simmons [2]).

Appendix A
Material properties of fluids

Temperature (°C)	Density, ρ (g/cm^3)	Viscosity, μ (g/cm per s)	Thermal conductivity, k (erg/cm per s °C)	Heat capacity, C_p (cm^2/°C per s^2)
Water/physiologic saline[a]				
20	0.9985	0.01000	5.98×10^4	4.181×10^7
25	0.997	0.00904	6.06×10^4	4.180×10^7
30	0.9955	0.00818	6.14×10^4	4.179×10^7
35	0.994	0.00727	6.22×10^4	4.179×10^7
37	0.993	0.00692	6.25×10^4	4.178×10^7
40	0.992	0.00640	6.30×10^4	4.178×10^7
Air				
20	0.00120	1.82×10^{-4}	2.57×10^3	1.005×10^7
25	0.00118	1.85×10^{-4}	2.60×10^3	1.005×10^7
30	0.00116	1.87×10^{-4}	2.64×10^3	1.005×10^7
35	0.00114	1.89×10^{-4}	2.67×10^3	1.005×10^7
37	0.00114	1.90×10^{-4}	2.68×10^3	1.005×10^7
40	0.00113	1.91×10^{-4}	2.70×10^3	1.005×10^7
Blood				
37	1.05–1.06	0.03–0.04	$(4.9–5.1) \times 10^4$	3.6×10^7
Plasma				
37	1.022–1.026	0.011–0.013	$(5.7–5.9) \times 10^4$	3.9×10^7

[a] The density of physiologic saline is 1.0067 times that of water.

Temperature (°C)	Surface tension, σ (dyne/cm)
Water/air	
20	72.8
25	72
30	71.2
35	70.4
37	70.1
40	69.6

Appendix B
Transport equations

The continuity equation (mass conservation)

$$\frac{\mathscr{D}\rho}{\mathscr{D}t} = -\rho \nabla \cdot \mathbf{v}$$

(Note that, when the density is constant, the continuity equation reduces to $\nabla \cdot \mathbf{v} = 0$.)

For Cartesian coordinates (x, y, z), with velocity components $\mathbf{v} = (v_x, v_y, v_z)$:

$$\frac{\partial \rho}{\partial t} + \frac{\partial(\rho v_x)}{\partial x} + \frac{\partial(\rho v_y)}{\partial y} + \frac{\partial(\rho v_z)}{\partial z} = 0$$

For cylindrical polar coordinates (r, θ, z), with velocity components $\mathbf{v} = (v_r, v_\theta, v_z)$:

$$\frac{\partial \rho}{\partial t} + \frac{1}{r}\frac{\partial}{\partial r}(\rho r v_r) + \frac{1}{r}\frac{\partial(\rho v_\theta)}{\partial \theta} + \frac{\partial(\rho v_z)}{\partial z} = 0$$

For spherical coordinates (r, θ, ϕ), with velocity components $\mathbf{v} = (v_r, v_\theta, v_\phi)$ $(0 < \theta < \pi, 0 < \phi < 2\pi)$:

$$\frac{\partial \rho}{\partial t} + \frac{1}{r^2}\frac{\partial}{\partial r}(\rho r^2 v_r) + \frac{1}{r \sin \theta}\frac{\partial(\rho v_\theta \sin \theta)}{\partial \theta} + \frac{1}{r \sin \theta}\frac{\partial(\rho v_\phi)}{\partial \phi} = 0$$

The Navier–Stokes equations (incompressible, constant viscosity, body force/mass = g)

$$\rho\frac{\mathscr{D}\mathbf{v}}{\mathscr{D}t} = -\nabla p + \mu \nabla^2 \mathbf{v} + \rho \mathbf{g}$$

For Cartesian coordinates (x, y, z), with velocity components $\mathbf{v} = (v_x, v_y, v_z)$:

$$x\text{-direction: } \rho \frac{\mathscr{D} v_x}{\mathscr{D} t} = -\frac{\partial p}{\partial x} + \mu \nabla^2 v_x + \rho g_x$$

$$y\text{-direction: } \rho \frac{\mathscr{D} v_y}{\mathscr{D} t} = -\frac{\partial p}{\partial y} + \mu \nabla^2 v_y + \rho g_y$$

$$z\text{-direction: } \rho \frac{\mathscr{D} v_z}{\mathscr{D} t} = -\frac{\partial p}{\partial z} + \mu \nabla^2 v_z + \rho g_z$$

For cylindrical polar coordinates (r, θ, z), with velocity components $\mathbf{v} = (v_r, v_\theta, v_z)$:

$$r\text{-direction: } \rho \frac{\mathscr{D} v_r}{\mathscr{D} t} - \frac{\rho}{r} v_\theta^2 = -\frac{\partial p}{\partial r} + \mu \left(\nabla^2 v_r - \frac{v_r}{r^2} - \frac{2}{r^2} \frac{\partial v_\theta}{\partial \theta} \right) + \rho g_r$$

$$\theta\text{-direction: } \rho \frac{\mathscr{D} v_\theta}{\mathscr{D} t} + \frac{\rho}{r} v_r v_\theta = -\frac{1}{r} \frac{\partial p}{\partial \theta} + \mu \left(\nabla^2 v_\theta - \frac{v_\theta}{r^2} + \frac{2}{r^2} \frac{\partial v_r}{\partial \theta} \right) + \rho g_\theta$$

$$z\text{-direction: } \rho \frac{\mathscr{D} v_z}{\mathscr{D} t} = -\frac{\partial p}{\partial z} + \mu \nabla^2 v_z + \rho g_z$$

For spherical coordinates (r, θ, ϕ), with velocity components $\mathbf{v} = (v_r, v_\theta, v_\phi)$ $(0 < \theta < \pi, 0 < \phi < 2\pi)$:

r-direction:

$$\rho \frac{\mathscr{D} v_r}{\mathscr{D} t} - \frac{\rho}{r} \left(v_\theta^2 + v_\phi^2 \right) = -\frac{\partial p}{\partial r} + \mu \left(\nabla^2 v_r - \frac{2 v_r}{r^2} - \frac{2}{r^2} \frac{\partial v_\theta}{\partial \theta} - \frac{2 v_\theta \cot \theta}{r^2} - \frac{2}{r^2 \sin \theta} \frac{\partial v_\phi}{\partial \phi} \right)$$
$$+ \rho g_r$$

θ-direction:

$$\rho \frac{\mathscr{D} v_\theta}{\mathscr{D} t} + \frac{\rho}{r} \left(v_r v_\theta - v_\phi^2 \cot \theta \right) = -\frac{1}{r} \frac{\partial p}{\partial \theta}$$
$$+ \mu \left(\nabla^2 v_\theta + \frac{2}{r^2} \frac{\partial v_r}{\partial \theta} - \frac{v_\theta}{r^2 \sin^2 \theta} - \frac{2 \cos \theta}{r^2 \sin^2 \theta} \frac{\partial v_\phi}{\partial \phi} \right)$$
$$+ \rho g_\theta$$

ϕ-direction:

$$\rho \frac{\mathscr{D} v_\phi}{\mathscr{D} t} + \frac{\rho}{r} \left(v_r v_\phi + v_\theta v_\phi \cot \theta \right) = -\frac{1}{r \sin \theta} \frac{\partial p}{\partial \phi}$$
$$+ \mu \left(\nabla^2 v_\phi + \frac{2}{r^2 \sin^2 \theta} \frac{\partial v_r}{\partial \phi} + \frac{2 \cos \theta}{r^2 \sin \theta} \frac{\partial v_\phi}{\partial \phi} - \frac{v_\phi}{r^2 \sin^2 \theta} \right)$$
$$+ \rho g_\phi$$

The convection–diffusion equation (constant D, dilute limit)

$$\frac{\mathscr{D}C}{\mathscr{D}t} = D\,\nabla^2 C + \dot{\varepsilon}$$

The energy equation (constant k)

$$\rho C_p \frac{\mathscr{D}T}{\mathscr{D}t} = k\,\nabla^2 T + \dot{q}$$

The Laplacian of a scalar

For Cartesian coordinates (x, y, z):

$$\nabla^2 f = \frac{\partial^2 f}{\partial x^2} + \frac{\partial^2 f}{\partial y^2} + \frac{\partial^2 f}{\partial z^2}$$

For cylindrical polar coordinates (r, θ, z):

$$\nabla^2 f = \frac{1}{r}\frac{\partial}{\partial r}\left(r\frac{\partial f}{\partial r}\right) + \frac{1}{r^2}\frac{\partial f}{\partial \theta^2} + \frac{\partial^2 f}{\partial z^2}$$

For spherical coordinates (r, θ, ϕ) $(0 < \theta < \pi, 0 < \phi < 2\pi)$:

$$\nabla^2 f = \frac{1}{r^2}\frac{\partial}{\partial r}\left(r^2\frac{\partial f}{\partial r}\right) + \frac{1}{r^2 \sin\theta}\frac{\partial}{\partial \theta}\left(\sin\theta\frac{\partial f}{\partial \theta}\right) + \frac{1}{r^2 \sin^2\theta}\frac{\partial^2 f}{\partial \phi^2}$$

The substantive/substantial/Lagrangian derivative

$$\frac{\mathscr{D}f}{\mathscr{D}t} = \frac{\partial f}{\partial t} + \mathbf{v}\cdot\nabla f$$

For Cartesian coordinates (x, y, z), with velocity components $\mathbf{v} = (v_x, v_y, v_z)$:

$$\frac{\mathscr{D}f}{\mathscr{D}t} = \frac{\partial f}{\partial t} + v_x \frac{\partial f}{\partial x} + v_y \frac{\partial f}{\partial y} + v_z \frac{\partial f}{\partial z}$$

For cylindrical polar coordinates (r, θ, z), with velocity components $\mathbf{v} = (v_r, v_\theta, v_z)$:

$$\frac{\mathscr{D}f}{\mathscr{D}t} = \frac{\partial f}{\partial t} + v_r \frac{\partial f}{\partial t} + \frac{v_\theta}{r} \frac{\partial f}{\partial \theta} + v_z \frac{\partial f}{\partial z}$$

For spherical coordinates (r, θ, ϕ), with velocity components $\mathbf{v} = (v_r, v_\theta, v_\phi)$ $(0 < \theta < \pi, 0 < \phi < 2\pi)$:

$$\frac{\mathscr{D}f}{\mathscr{D}t} = \frac{\partial f}{\partial t} + v_r \frac{\partial f}{\partial r} + \frac{v_\theta}{r} \frac{\partial f}{\partial \theta} + \frac{v_\phi}{r \sin \theta} \frac{\partial f}{\partial \phi}$$

Appendix C
Charts

We present here several charts that are useful to the solution of some of the problems in this text.

The error function

The error function is useful for the solution of fluid-mechanics problems (e.g. the Rayleigh problem) and those involving transient mass and heat transfer:

$$\text{erf}(z) = \frac{2}{\sqrt{\pi}} \int_0^z e^{-t^2}\, dt$$

$$\text{erfc}(z) = 1 - \text{erf}(z)$$

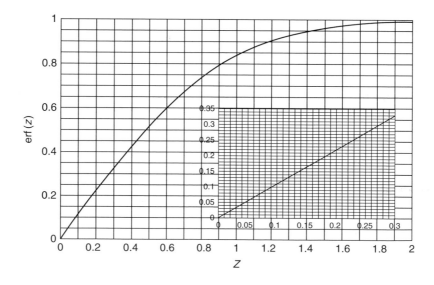

Transient mass and heat conduction

We consider here the unsteady diffusion of mass, or equivalently the conduction of heat, within four objects: a slab (of thickness $2L$), a cylinder (of radius L), a sphere (of radius L), and a semi-infinite wall ($x > 0$). We consider the first three objects as a group, and then consider the semi-infinite wall. We consider the case in which the object is at uniform initial temperature $T_{initial}$ (for heat transfer) or contains a species at uniform initial concentration $C_{initial}$ (for mass transfer) and is placed in a fluid with constant temperature T_∞ or concentration C_∞ at time $t = 0$. The charts show the dimensionless concentration or dimensionless temperature

$$\Theta = \frac{C(t) - C_\infty}{C_{initial} - C_\infty} = \frac{T(t) - T_\infty}{T_{initial} - T_\infty}$$

as a function of two dimensionless variables: the Fourier number Fo (dimensionless time) and the Biot number Bi:

$$Fo = \frac{Dt}{L^2} \quad \text{or} \quad Fo = \frac{\alpha t}{L^2}$$

and

$$Bi = \frac{hL}{D} \quad \text{or} \quad Bi = \frac{hL}{k}$$

where D is the diffusion coefficient of the species (mass transfer), α is the thermal diffusivity (heat transfer), h is the mass- or heat-transfer coefficient at the surface, and k is the thermal conductivity (heat transfer). Here $\alpha = k/(\rho C_p)$, where ρ is the density of the object and C_p is its heat capacity (at constant pressure). The mass or heat transfer coefficient is defined in terms of the mass (j) or heat flux (q) leaving the surface of the object:

$$j = q = h(C_{surface} - C_\infty) = h(T_{surface} - T_\infty)$$

The solutions to these problems are given in Carslaw and Jaeger [17].
For the slab ($-L < x < L$)

$$\Theta = \sum_{n=1}^{\infty} \frac{2Bi \exp(-\alpha_n^2 Fo)\cos(\alpha_n x/L)}{[Bi(Bi + 1) + \alpha_n^2]\cos(\alpha_n)}$$

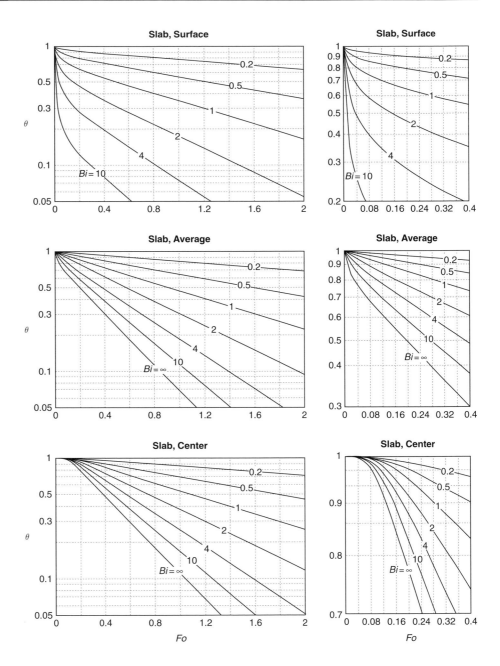

where α_n are roots of the equation $\alpha_n \tan \alpha_n = Bi$. The first six roots of this equation are tabulated in Carslaw and Jaeger [17]. The chart above shows these solutions.

For the cylinder ($r < L$)

$$\Theta = \sum_{n=1}^{\infty} \frac{2Bi \exp(-\beta_n^2 Fo)J_0(\beta_n r/L)}{(Bi^2 + \beta_n^2)J_0(\beta_n)}$$

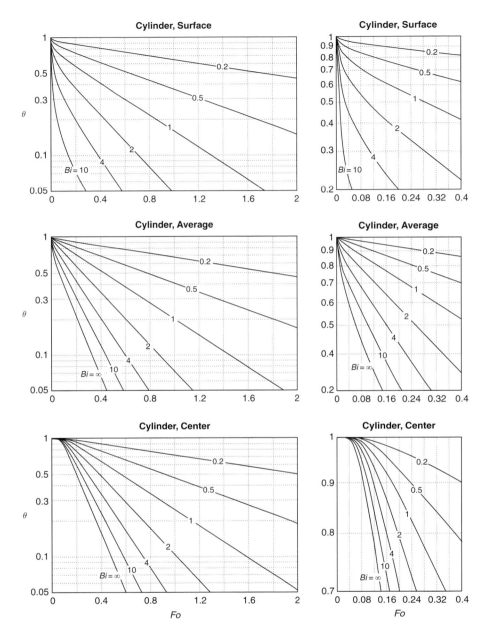

where β_n are roots of the equation $\beta_n J_1(\beta_n)/J_0(\beta_n) = Bi$. The first six roots of this equation are tabulated in Carslaw and Jaeger [17]. The chart above shows these solutions.

For the sphere $(r < L)$

$$\Theta = \sum_{n=1}^{\infty} \frac{2Bi\left[(Bi-1)^2 + \beta_n^2\right]\exp(-\gamma_n^2 Fo)\sin(\gamma_n r/L)\sin(\gamma_n)}{\gamma_n^2\left[Bi(Bi-1) + \gamma_n^2\right]r/L}$$

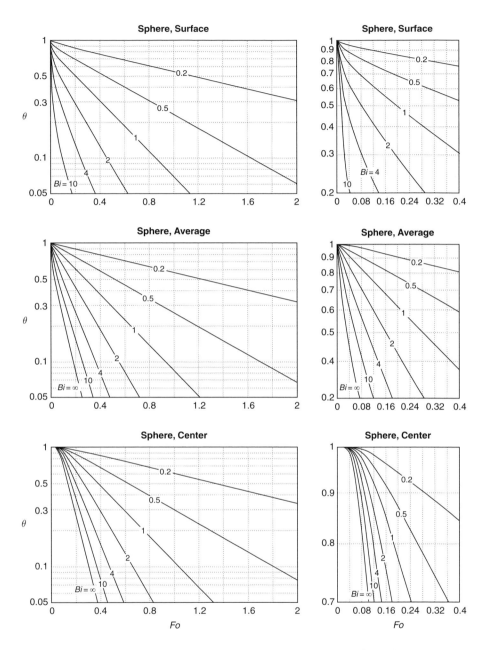

where γ_n are roots of the equation $\gamma_n \cot \gamma_n = 1 - Bi$. The first six roots of this equation are tabulated in Carslaw and Jaeger [17]. The chart above shows these solutions.

In the case of a semi-infinite wall with a heat or mass transfer coefficient specified at $x = 0$, the definitions of the Fourier number and Biot number become

$$Fo = \frac{Dt}{x^2} \quad \text{or} \quad Fo = \frac{\alpha t}{x^2}$$

and

$$Bi = \frac{hx}{D} \quad \text{or} \quad Bi = \frac{hx}{k}$$

Then [18],

$$\Theta = \text{erf}\left(\frac{1}{2\sqrt{Fo}}\right) + \exp(Bi + Bi^2 Fo)\left[1 - \text{erf}\left(Bi\sqrt{Fo} + \frac{1}{2\sqrt{Fo}}\right)\right]$$

A chart of the error function was shown earlier in this appendix. Note that in the case where the surface temperature is specified ($Bi = \infty$), this equation reduces to

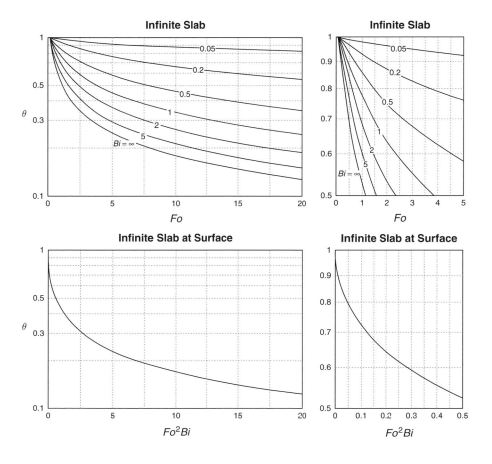

$$\Theta = \mathrm{erf}\left(\frac{1}{2\sqrt{Fo}}\right)$$

Note also that, at $x = 0$, the equation becomes

$$\Theta = \exp(Bi^2 Fo)\left[1 - \mathrm{erf}\left(Bi\sqrt{Fo}\right)\right]$$

These relations are plotted in the final set of figures.

References

[1]   Sonin, A. A. and Shapiro, A. H., *Advanced Fluid Mechanics Problems*, 1986, Cambridge, MA: Massachusetts Institute of Technology.

[2]   Ethier, C. R. and Simmons, C. A., *Introductory Biomechanics: From Cells to Organisms*, 2007, Cambridge: Cambridge University Press.

[3]   Hale, J. F., McDonald, D. A., and Womersley, J. R., Velocity profiles of oscillating arterial flow, with some calculations of viscous drag and the Reynolds number. *Journal of Physiology – London*, 1955. 128:629–640.

[4]   Gray, H. *Anatomy of the Human Body*, 1918, Philadelphia, PA: Lea & Febiger.

[5]   Rosendahl, L., Using a multi-parameter particle shape description to predict the motion of non-spherical particle shapes in swirling flow. *Applied Mathematical Modelling*, 2000. 24:11–25.

[6]   Huggert, A., An experiment in determining the pore size distribution curve to the filtration angle of the eye. *Acta Ophthalmologica*, 1957. 35:12–19, 105–112.

[7]   Jouan-Hureaux, V., Audonnet-Blaise, S., Lacatusu, D. *et al.*, Effects of a new perfluorocarbon emulsion on human plasma and whole-blood viscosity in the presence of albumin, hydroxyethyl starch, or modified fluid gelatin: an *in vitro* rheologic approach. *Transfusion*, 2006. 46:1892–1898.

[8]   Barbee, J. H. and Cokelet, G. R., The Fåhræus effect. *Microvascular Research*, 1971. 3:6–16.

[9]   Kynch, G. J., The effective viscosity of suspensions of spherical particles. *Proceedings of the Royal Society of London Series A – Mathematical and Physical Sciences*, 1956. 237:90–116.

[10] Henry, R. R., Mudaliar, S. R. D., Howland, W. C. III *et al.*, Inhaled insulin using the AERx Insulin Diabetes Management System in healthy and asthmatic subjects. *Diabetes Care*, 2003. 26:764–769.

[11] Scharrer, E., The blood vessels of the nervous system. *Quarterly Review of Biology*, 1944. 19:308–318.

[12] Lin, C.-W., Wang, W., Challa, P., Epstein, D. L., and Yuan, F., Transscleral diffusion of ethacrynic acid and sodium fluorescein. *Molecular Vision*, 2007. 13:243–251.

[13] Bird, R. B., Stewart, W. E., and Lightfoot, E. N., *Transport Phenomena*. Revised 2nd ed. 2006, New York, NY: John Wiley & Sons.

[14] Yang, M. C. and Cussler, E. L., Designing hollow-fiber contactors. *AIChE Journal*, 1986. 32:1910–1916.

[15] Yang, M. C. and Cussler, E. L., Artificial gills. *Journal of Membrane Science*, 1989. 42:273–284.

[16] Landis, E. M., Micro-injection studies of capillary permeability II. The relation between capillary pressure and the rate at which fluid passes through the walls of single capillaries. *American Journal of Physiology*, 1927. 82:217–238.

[17] Carslaw, H. S. and Jaeger, J. C., *Conduction of Heat in Solids*, 1959, Oxford: Oxford University Press.

[18] Welty, J., Wicks, C., and Wilson, R., *Fundamentals of Momentum, Heat and Mass Transfer*, 1969, New York, NY: John Wiley & Sons.

[19] Gradshteyn, I. S. and Ryzhik, I. M. *Table of Integrals, Series, and Products*, 1965, New York, NY: Academic Press, formula 3.661.4.

Permissions

Chapter 3, Problem 3.12: copyright and permission from the Massachusetts Institute of Technology.

Chapter 5, Problem 5.4: copyright and permission from John Wiley & Sons, Inc.

Chapter 8, Problem 8.9: copyright and permission from Elsevier.

Chapter 15, Problem 15.6: copyright and permission from John Wiley & Sons, Inc.